CONTENTS

Chapter 1: Introduction	1
Chapter 2: Etiology and Risk Factors	20
Chapter 3: Pathogenesis and Molecular Mechanisms	45
Chapter 4: Clinical Presentation and Diagnosis	76
Chapter 5: Treatment Approaches	108
Chapter 6: Prognosis and Survival	139
Chapter 7: Thymic Tumors in Pediatrics	170
Chapter 8: Holistic Health and Well-Being	202
Chapter 9: Advances in Imaging and Diagnostics	235
Chapter 10: Targeted Therapies and Precision Medicine	268
Chapter 11: Experimental Models and Basic Research	301
Chapter 12: Global Perspectives and Future Directions	338

CHAPTER 1: INTRODUCTION

The thymus, a seemingly unassuming organ nestled in the mediastinum, plays a profound and intricate role in the orchestration of the immune system. Often overlooked, it harbors secrets both of profound importance and complexity. Within its compact structure, the thymus shapes and molds the T lymphocytes, the vigilant guardians of our immune defenses, equipping them with the knowledge and wisdom to distinguish friend from foe.

However, amidst the intricate dance of immunity, a dark specter can arise – the malignant neoplasm of the thymus. In this treatise, we embark on a comprehensive journey into the realm of thymic tumors, delving deep into the labyrinthine pathways of medicine, biochemistry, anatomy, and holistic health.

This treatise endeavors to be a guiding beacon for clinicians, researchers, and all those who seek to understand and combat this enigmatic foe. Through its pages, we shall traverse the landscape of etiology, where genetic predispositions, environmental influences, and intricate molecular mechanisms converge to instigate disease. We will explore the clinical presentation, diagnosis, and the ever-evolving arsenal of treatment strategies that seek to restore harmony within the mediastinum.

But our journey extends beyond the conventional boundaries

of medicine. We shall also illuminate the holistic health aspects, recognizing the patient as a whole, not merely as a bearer of tumors, but as a soul seeking healing, both physically and emotionally. Nutrition, exercise, and mindfulness shall find their rightful place in our discourse.

Moreover, we shall peer into the future, where advanced imaging, precision medicine, and global collaborations hold the promise of better outcomes for those afflicted by thymic tumors. Through the collective efforts of researchers, healthcare providers, and advocates, we aspire to envision a world where thymic malignancies no longer cast their ominous shadows.

As we embark on this expedition into the intricate world of malignant neoplasm of the thymus, we invite you to join us in this pursuit of knowledge, understanding, and hope. The thymus, though often overlooked, is a remarkable organ, and the study of its malignancies unveils both the complexity of nature and the resilience of human endeavor.

May this treatise serve as a testament to our dedication to unraveling the mysteries of the thymus and advancing the care and well-being of those impacted by these formidable adversaries.

1.1 Definition and Overview of Malignant Neoplasm of the Thymus

Malignant neoplasm of the thymus, commonly referred to as thymic cancer or thymoma, represents a group of rare and intricate malignancies arising from the thymus gland, a vital component of the immune system. The thymus, though relatively small in adulthood, plays a pivotal role in the development and maturation of T lymphocytes, a type of white blood cell essential for adaptive immune responses.

Anatomy and Function of the Thymus: The thymus is a bi-lobed organ situated in the anterior mediastinum, just behind the breastbone (sternum). It is most active during childhood and adolescence, gradually diminishing in size and activity as one ages. The primary function of the thymus is to educate and train immature T cells, guiding them through a selection process that ensures they recognize and respond to foreign pathogens while avoiding harmful reactions against self-tissues.

Types of Thymic Tumors: Malignant neoplasms of the thymus encompass a spectrum of tumor types, with thymomas and thymic carcinomas being the most common. Thymomas are typically slow-growing and tend to maintain some aspects of thymic tissue structure, while thymic carcinomas are more aggressive and lack this organization. Other rare types of thymic tumors may include neuroendocrine tumors, lymphomas, and sarcomas.

Clinical Significance: Thymic malignancies are rare, accounting for only a small fraction of all cancers. They can manifest with a wide range of symptoms, including chest pain, cough, shortness of breath, and myasthenia gravis, a neuromuscular disorder often associated with thymic tumors. Due to their location in the mediastinum, thymic cancers can also exert pressure on nearby structures, leading to various clinical presentations.

Diagnostic Challenges: Diagnosing thymic tumors can be complex, requiring a combination of imaging studies (such as CT scans and MRI), histopathological examination of tissue samples obtained through biopsy, and sometimes molecular analysis. The rarity and heterogeneity of these tumors can pose challenges in accurate diagnosis.

Prognosis and Treatment: The prognosis for patients

with malignant neoplasm of the thymus varies widely depending on factors like tumor type, stage, and histological characteristics. Treatment options may include surgery, radiation therapy, chemotherapy, targeted therapies, and immunotherapies, often used in combination to achieve the best outcomes.

Understanding the intricacies of malignant neoplasm of the thymus is essential for clinicians and researchers alike. This treatise will delve deeper into the nuances of these tumors, exploring their etiology, molecular mechanisms, diagnosis, treatment, and the holistic care of individuals facing this challenging disease.

1.2 Historical Perspective and Epidemiology

The historical journey of understanding malignant neoplasms of the thymus, commonly referred to as thymic cancers, is a testament to the evolution of medical knowledge and the enduring pursuit of unraveling the mysteries of these rare malignancies. This section will explore the historical perspective of thymic tumors and provide a comprehensive overview of their epidemiology.

Historical Perspective:

The history of thymic tumors is intertwined with the broader history of thymus gland exploration. Here, we trace the milestones and notable discoveries that have shaped our understanding of these intriguing neoplasms.

1. **Ancient Recognition:** The thymus, though not fully understood, has been recognized since ancient times. It was mentioned by the ancient Greeks, who referred to it as the "seat of the soul" due to its prominent location in the chest. However, its function remained a mystery.
2. **Thymus Function:** The actual function of the

thymus as a critical organ for immune system development was not elucidated until the early 20th century. In 1961, Jacques Miller and Jill O'Farrell provided groundbreaking evidence of its role in T-cell development in a landmark study.
3. **Emergence of Thymic Tumors:** As our understanding of the thymus evolved, so did our recognition of thymic tumors. The term "thymoma" was coined in the mid-20th century to describe the most common type of thymic tumor.
4. **Myasthenia Gravis Connection:** The association between thymic tumors and myasthenia gravis (MG), a neuromuscular disorder, was established in the 20th century. The removal of thymic tumors often leads to symptom improvement in MG patients.
5. **Advances in Surgical Techniques:** Surgical management of thymic tumors advanced significantly in the latter half of the 20th century, with the development of techniques such as median sternotomy and minimally invasive procedures.
6. **Evolving Treatment Paradigms:** Over the past few decades, treatment options for thymic tumors have expanded to include radiation therapy, chemotherapy, targeted therapies, and immunotherapies, reflecting advancements in oncology.
7. **Current Research:** Ongoing research aims to understand the molecular underpinnings of thymic tumors, identify novel therapeutic targets, and improve the overall prognosis for affected individuals.

Epidemiology:

Understanding the epidemiology of thymic tumors is essential to grasp the broader impact of these rare cancers on public health. While thymic tumors are relatively uncommon, their incidence, demographics, and associated factors provide valuable insights.

1. **Incidence:** Thymic tumors are rare, accounting for approximately 0.2% to 1.5% of all malignancies. The annual incidence varies by region but is generally estimated to be around 1 to 3 cases per million people.
2. **Age and Gender:** Thymic tumors often manifest in adults aged 40 to 60 years, but they can occur at any age. They are slightly more common in men than in women.
3. **Geographical Variation:** The incidence of thymic tumors varies globally. Some regions, such as Asia, have reported higher incidences, possibly due to genetic factors or differences in diagnostic practices.
4. **Myasthenia Gravis Association:** Myasthenia gravis is found in approximately 30% to 50% of thymoma cases, highlighting a strong association between these conditions.
5. **Histological Types:** Thymomas are the most common thymic tumors, representing about 90% of cases. Thymic carcinomas are rarer but tend to be more aggressive.
6. **Tumor Staging:** Thymic tumors are often classified using the Masaoka-Koga staging system, which considers factors such as tumor invasion into surrounding structures and lymph node involvement.
7. **Survival Rates:** The prognosis for thymic tumors varies widely depending on factors like histology and stage. Overall, thymomas tend to have a more favorable prognosis than thymic carcinomas. The 5-year survival rate for thymomas is around 90%, whereas it is lower for thymic carcinomas, at approximately 50% to 60%.
8. **Treatment Outcomes:** Advances in treatment have improved outcomes for many patients. Surgical resection remains a cornerstone of treatment, often combined with adjuvant therapies.

9. **Rare Subtypes:** Other rare thymic tumor subtypes, such as thymic neuroendocrine tumors and lymphomas, exhibit distinct epidemiological patterns.
10. **Future Trends:** As research continues, efforts to better understand the epidemiology of thymic tumors will help refine diagnostic and treatment strategies, ultimately improving patient outcomes.

In summary, the historical perspective of thymic tumors reflects the gradual unfolding of knowledge about the thymus and its associated malignancies. While these tumors are rare, their epidemiological characteristics offer valuable insights for clinicians, researchers, and policymakers working to address the challenges posed by thymic cancers.

1.3 Anatomy of the Thymus Gland

The thymus gland, often described as the "master of immunity," is a remarkable organ nestled in the anterior mediastinum of the chest. Despite its relatively small size, the thymus plays an outsized role in the development and maturation of T lymphocytes, a critical component of the immune system. In this section, we will explore the anatomy of the thymus gland, delving into its structure, location, development, and its pivotal role in immune function.

Location and Gross Anatomy:

The thymus is a bilobed organ, meaning it consists of two distinct lobes or halves. It is situated in the anterior mediastinum, a region within the thoracic cavity, just behind the sternum (breastbone). The location of the thymus makes it particularly accessible for surgical procedures when necessary.

Each lobe of the thymus is pyramidal in shape and is approximately 5-7 centimeters in length in adults. The two lobes are connected by an isthmus, a bridge of thymic tissue.

The thymus gland tends to be more prominent and active during childhood and adolescence, gradually decreasing in size and activity as individuals age.

Microscopic Anatomy:

To truly appreciate the complexity of the thymus, one must venture into its microscopic world, where immune cells are molded and educated to defend the body against pathogens.

1. **Thymic Lobules:** Each thymic lobe is divided into numerous lobules. Within these lobules, the thymus houses a highly specialized microenvironment that supports T cell development.
2. **Cortex and Medulla:** Thymic lobules are further divided into two distinct regions: the cortex and the medulla. These regions play crucial roles in T cell maturation.
    - *Cortex:* The cortex is the outer layer of each thymic lobule. It is densely populated with immature T cells, or thymocytes, at various stages of development. Here, thymocytes undergo positive and negative selection processes, ensuring that they can recognize foreign antigens without attacking the body's own tissues.
    - *Medulla:* Deeper within each lobule lies the medulla. This region contains fewer thymocytes but is crucial for further T cell maturation. It is here that self-tolerance is reinforced, ensuring that T cells do not attack the body's own cells and tissues.
3. **Thymic Epithelial Cells (TECs):** TECs are the stromal cells of the thymus and are indispensable for T cell development. They provide critical signals to thymocytes, guiding their maturation. TECs also play a

role in central tolerance by presenting self-antigens to thymocytes, helping to eliminate potentially harmful autoreactive T cells.
4. **Hassall's Corpuscles:** These are unique structures found in the medulla of the thymus and consist of concentric layers of epithelial cells. Their exact function is not fully understood, but they are thought to be involved in mediating immune tolerance.

Development and Function:

The thymus gland is particularly active during the early stages of life and childhood. Its development and function can be summarized as follows:

1. **Embryonic Development:** The thymus develops from the third pharyngeal pouch, which is a structure in the embryonic throat region. It arises from the endodermal tissue and migrates to its final location in the anterior mediastinum.
2. **Maturation of T Cells:** The primary function of the thymus is the maturation of T lymphocytes. It is within the thymus that T cell precursors, known as thymocytes, undergo a rigorous process of education and selection. This process ensures that T cells are capable of recognizing foreign antigens while remaining tolerant to self-antigens.
3. **Positive and Negative Selection:** Thymocytes in the cortex are exposed to self-antigens presented by thymic epithelial cells (TECs). Those that bind too weakly or too strongly to self-antigens undergo either positive selection (to ensure antigen recognition) or negative selection (to eliminate autoreactive cells), respectively.
4. **Migration of Mature T Cells:** Once T cells have successfully completed their education and selection processes within the thymus, they migrate to

secondary lymphoid organs such as the lymph nodes and spleen, where they play vital roles in immune responses.
5. **Involution with Age:** The thymus reaches its maximum size during puberty but begins to involute (shrink) with age. This involution is accompanied by a decline in thymic function, which can impact immune responses, particularly in older individuals.

Clinical Relevance:

Understanding the anatomy and function of the thymus is of paramount importance in the context of thymic tumors. Thymomas and thymic carcinomas, the most common thymic malignancies, can disrupt the normal architecture and function of the thymus. Surgical interventions and treatments for thymic tumors must carefully consider preserving thymic function and minimizing disruption to the immune system.

In conclusion, the thymus gland, with its unique anatomy and pivotal role in immune function, stands as a testament to the intricacies of the human body. While its significance may wane with age, its legacy persists in the T cells that it educates and sends forth to protect the body against pathogens and maintain immune tolerance. Understanding the anatomy of the thymus is not only vital for appreciating its role in health but also for addressing the challenges posed by thymic tumors and their impact on immune function.

1.4 Thymic Development and Function

The thymus, a seemingly unassuming organ nestled in the chest, holds a pivotal role in the intricate symphony of the immune system. Its development and function are nothing short of remarkable, as it serves as both a school and a boot camp for T lymphocytes, critical components of the adaptive immune response. In this section, we will delve deep into the fascinating world of thymic development and function, exploring the intricate processes that shape the immune system's warriors.

Thymic Development:

The development of the thymus, like many biological processes, begins in the embryonic stages of life. Understanding its embryological origins provides insights into its structure and function.

1. **Origins:** The thymus has a complex embryonic origin. It arises from the third pharyngeal pouch, a structure in the throat region of the developing embryo. The third pouch gives rise to the thymus, while other pharyngeal pouches contribute to the development of other structures, such as the parathyroid glands.
2. **Migration:** After its initial formation, the thymus migrates from its embryonic location to the anterior mediastinum, where it will reside throughout life. This migration is facilitated by a series of intricate molecular signals and interactions.
3. **Maturation:** As the thymus reaches its final destination in the chest, it continues to mature. It differentiates into distinct regions, such as the cortex and medulla, each with specialized functions in T cell development and education.

Thymic Function:

The thymus is often likened to a "T cell university" where immature T lymphocytes, called thymocytes, undergo a rigorous educational process. This process ensures that T cells can effectively recognize and respond to foreign antigens while avoiding self-reactivity.

1. **Positive Selection:** Positive selection is the first crucial step in thymocyte education. Thymocytes in the cortex of the thymus are exposed to a diverse array of self-antigens presented by thymic epithelial cells (TECs). Those thymocytes that can bind to self-antigens presented by major histocompatibility complexes (MHC) with moderate affinity receive a "survival signal." These positively selected thymocytes move on to the next phase of maturation.
2. **Negative Selection:** Negative selection is equally vital. Thymocytes that bind too strongly to self-antigens, indicating a high risk of autoimmunity, undergo apoptosis (cell death) in the cortex. This process eliminates autoreactive T cells, preventing them from causing harm to the body's own tissues.
3. **Migration to the Medulla:** After passing positive and negative selection in the cortex, thymocytes move to the medulla, the inner region of the thymus. Here, they encounter an even wider range of self-antigens presented by medullary thymic epithelial cells (mTECs). This reinforces self-tolerance and ensures that T cells do not attack the body's own tissues.
4. **T Cell Receptor Rearrangement:** During their time in the thymus, thymocytes undergo a process called T cell receptor (TCR) rearrangement. This genetic reshuffling results in diverse TCRs, enabling T cells to recognize a vast array of antigens.
5. **Exit from the Thymus:** Only thymocytes that successfully complete their education, having passed both positive and negative selection, are allowed to exit the thymus and enter the bloodstream as mature T cells. These T cells are equipped with TCRs capable of recognizing specific antigens presented by MHC molecules.

The Role of Thymic Epithelial Cells (TECs):

Thymic epithelial cells (TECs) are the unsung heroes of thymic development and function. They serve as the educators, presenting self-antigens to thymocytes and shaping their destiny.

1. **TEC Subtypes:** TECs can be divided into two primary subtypes: cortical TECs (cTECs) and medullary TECs (mTECs). cTECs are mainly involved in positive selection, presenting self-antigens to thymocytes in the cortex. mTECs, on the other hand, are central to negative selection, presenting a broader array of self-antigens in the medulla.
2. **Autoimmune Regulator (AIRE):** mTECs play a unique role in the induction of immune tolerance. They express a protein called Autoimmune Regulator (AIRE), which enables them to present a wide range of tissue-specific antigens. This process helps eliminate autoreactive T cells, preventing autoimmune diseases.

Clinical Relevance:

Understanding the development and function of the thymus has profound clinical implications. Thymic tumors, such as thymomas and thymic carcinomas, can disrupt the normal architecture and function of the thymus. Surgical interventions to remove these tumors must carefully consider preserving thymic function, especially in pediatric cases where the thymus is still actively educating T cells.

Additionally, age-related thymic involution, where the thymus gradually decreases in size and activity, can impact the immune system's ability to generate new T cells. This has implications for the susceptibility to infections and the development of autoimmune diseases in older individuals.

In conclusion, the thymus is not merely a passive organ but a dynamic educator, molding T cells into defenders of the body. Its development from embryonic origins, coupled with the intricacies of positive and negative selection and the crucial role of thymic epithelial cells, underpin its vital function in immune system maturation. Understanding the thymus's role in shaping the immune response is fundamental to appreciating its significance in health and disease.

1.5 Classification of Thymic Tumors

Thymic tumors, a diverse group of neoplasms arising from the thymus gland, present a complex challenge to clinicians and pathologists. These tumors exhibit a wide range of histological subtypes, clinical behaviors, and molecular characteristics. Accurate classification is essential for appropriate treatment and prognosis. In this section, we will explore the classification of thymic tumors, examining the various subtypes and their clinical significance.

Overview of Thymic Tumors:

Thymic tumors can be broadly categorized into two main groups: thymomas and thymic carcinomas. Each of these groups contains several histological subtypes, adding to the complexity of classification. Understanding these classifications is crucial for diagnosis, treatment planning, and predicting patient outcomes.

Thymomas:

Thymomas are the most common type of thymic tumor, accounting for approximately 90% of cases. They are typically slow-growing and have a more favorable prognosis compared to thymic carcinomas.

World Health Organization (WHO) Classification of

Thymomas:

Thymomas are classified into several subtypes based on their histological features. The WHO classification system provides a framework for categorizing thymomas into distinct groups:

1. **Type A Thymoma:** Type A thymomas are characterized by a predominantly spindle cell appearance. They tend to be well-differentiated and have a low potential for invasiveness.
2. **Type AB Thymoma:** Type AB thymomas are a combination of spindle cells and epithelial cells. They are also considered relatively low-grade tumors.
3. **Type B1 Thymoma:** Type B1 thymomas are characterized by a predominantly lymphocyte-rich background with scattered epithelial cells. They are generally low-grade tumors.
4. **Type B2 Thymoma:** Type B2 thymomas have a mixed population of epithelial cells and lymphocytes. They are considered intermediate-grade tumors.
5. **Type B3 Thymoma:** Type B3 thymomas are predominantly composed of epithelial cells with minimal lymphocytic infiltration. They tend to be higher-grade tumors.
6. **Type C Thymoma:** Type C thymomas are considered the most aggressive among thymomas. They exhibit invasive characteristics and may have areas of necrosis or hemorrhage.

Thymic Carcinomas:

Thymic carcinomas are a less common but more aggressive subgroup of thymic tumors. They tend to have a higher potential for metastasis and a less favorable prognosis compared to thymomas.

Histological Subtypes of Thymic Carcinomas:

Thymic carcinomas can also be classified into different histological subtypes, although this classification is not as standardized as that of thymomas. Subtypes of thymic carcinomas include:

1. **Squamous Cell Carcinoma:** This subtype exhibits features of squamous cell differentiation and is one of the most common histological types of thymic carcinomas.
2. **Adenocarcinoma:** Thymic adenocarcinomas exhibit glandular differentiation and are characterized by the presence of gland-like structures.
3. **Neuroendocrine Carcinoma:** Thymic neuroendocrine carcinomas, including small cell and large cell neuroendocrine carcinomas, have neuroendocrine features and may be associated with the production of hormones.
4. **Undifferentiated Carcinoma:** This category includes tumors that lack specific differentiation features and may have a high degree of cellular atypia.
5. **Lymphoepithelioma-Like Carcinoma:** Rarely, thymic carcinomas may exhibit a lymphoepithelioma-like appearance, resembling certain nasopharyngeal carcinomas.

Mixed Thymomas:

In addition to the above classifications, mixed thymomas are a unique category. These tumors exhibit features of both thymoma and thymic carcinoma, making classification and treatment decisions challenging.

Clinical Significance of Classification:

The classification of thymic tumors is of utmost importance due to the significant implications it carries for patient management:

1. **Treatment Planning:** The classification of thymic tumors guides treatment decisions. Thymomas, especially low-grade types, may be treated with surgical resection alone, while thymic carcinomas often require more aggressive approaches, including surgery, radiation therapy, and chemotherapy.
2. **Prognosis:** The histological subtype of a thymic tumor is a strong predictor of patient prognosis. Generally, lower-grade thymomas have a more favorable outlook than higher-grade thymomas and thymic carcinomas.
3. **Metastatic Potential:** Thymic carcinomas, particularly those with neuroendocrine features, are associated with a higher risk of metastasis to distant organs, affecting the choice of treatment and follow-up strategies.
4. **Clinical Trials:** Accurate classification is essential for enrolling patients in clinical trials evaluating targeted therapies or immunotherapies. Understanding the specific subtype of a thymic tumor can help tailor treatment options.

Challenges in Classification:

Classifying thymic tumors can be challenging due to the variability in histological appearance and the potential for mixed histology. Additionally, the rarity of these tumors can lead to limited experience among pathologists and clinicians.

Emerging Molecular Classification:

In recent years, efforts have been made to complement histological classification with molecular characterization of thymic tumors. Molecular profiling can provide additional insights into tumor behavior and guide treatment decisions. For example, genetic alterations in thymic tumors, such as mutations in genes like TP53 and KIT, are being explored as potential therapeutic targets.

Conclusion:

The classification of thymic tumors is a complex endeavor, involving both histological and, increasingly, molecular considerations. Accurate classification is essential for determining treatment strategies, predicting patient outcomes, and guiding research efforts to improve the management of these rare and heterogeneous neoplasms. As our understanding of thymic tumors continues to evolve, so too will our ability to refine their classification and tailor treatments for better patient outcomes.

1.6 Objectives and Structure of the Treatise

In the quest to unravel the intricacies of malignant neoplasm of the thymus, a multifaceted journey unfolds. This treatise embarks on that expedition, driven by the desire to comprehensively explore the vast terrain of thymic tumors. This section outlines the objectives of this treatise and provides an overview of its structured framework, guiding you through the rich tapestry of knowledge that encompasses the realm of thymic malignancies.

Objectives:

1. **Comprehensive Understanding:** The primary objective of this treatise is to provide a comprehensive understanding of malignant neoplasm of the thymus. We aim to equip clinicians, researchers, and healthcare professionals with a deep knowledge base to enhance the diagnosis, treatment, and care of individuals affected by these rare malignancies.
2. **Multidisciplinary Approach:** Thymic tumors demand a multidisciplinary approach, encompassing fields such

as oncology, surgery, pathology, immunology, and more. This treatise strives to bridge these disciplines, fostering a holistic comprehension of the disease.

3. **Holistic Health:** Beyond the confines of traditional medical knowledge, we recognize the importance of holistic health in the well-being of patients. As such, this treatise will delve into aspects of nutrition, exercise, mental health, and patient support, acknowledging the patient as a whole, not merely as a bearer of tumors.

4. **Advancements and Future Directions:** The field of thymic malignancies is dynamic, with ongoing research, technological advancements, and emerging therapies. This treatise aims to stay current, providing insights into the latest developments and future directions in the diagnosis and treatment of thymic tumors.

5. **Patient Empowerment:** Knowledge is a powerful tool, and we aspire to empower patients and their caregivers with a deeper understanding of thymic malignancies. Through this empowerment, we aim to enhance patient engagement in their healthcare journey.

CHAPTER 2: ETIOLOGY AND RISK FACTORS

2.1 Genetic Predisposition and Familial Syndromes

Malignant neoplasm of the thymus, though rare, can sometimes be associated with genetic predisposition and familial syndromes. Understanding the genetic factors contributing to thymic tumors is vital not only for diagnosis but also for patient management, counseling, and the development of targeted therapies. In this section, we will explore genetic predisposition, familial syndromes, and their relevance to thymic malignancies.

Genetic Predisposition to Thymic Tumors:

While thymic tumors are typically sporadic, meaning they occur by chance, there is growing evidence to suggest that genetic factors can predispose certain individuals to these malignancies. These genetic predispositions are not as well-defined as those seen in some other cancers but warrant investigation.

1. **Association with Immunodeficiency Syndromes:** Some individuals with underlying immunodeficiency syndromes, such as DiGeorge syndrome or complete DiGeorge anomaly (22q11.2 deletion syndrome), have an increased risk of developing thymic tumors.

DiGeorge syndrome is characterized by congenital heart defects, immune system abnormalities, and thymic hypoplasia, which can predispose individuals to thymic malignancies.
2. **Genetic Mutations:** While no specific genetic mutations have been definitively linked to the development of thymic tumors, ongoing research is exploring the role of genetic alterations in these malignancies. Mutations in genes like TP53 and KIT have been observed in some thymic tumors, although their significance and contribution to tumorigenesis are not fully understood.
3. **Hereditary Cancer Syndromes:** Thymic tumors can rarely occur in the context of hereditary cancer syndromes. For example, individuals with multiple endocrine neoplasia type 1 (MEN1) syndrome have an increased risk of developing various tumors, including thymic carcinoids.
4. **Genetic Susceptibility:** It is possible that there are yet-to-be-identified genetic susceptibility factors that predispose certain individuals to thymic tumors. Large-scale genetic studies are ongoing to uncover potential genetic risk factors.

Familial Syndromes Associated with Thymic Tumors:

In some cases, thymic tumors have been reported in families, suggesting a hereditary component. Familial syndromes associated with thymic tumors include:

1. **Multiple Endocrine Neoplasia Type 1 (MEN1) Syndrome:** MEN1 syndrome is an autosomal dominant genetic disorder caused by mutations in the MEN1 gene. It is characterized by the development of tumors in multiple endocrine organs, including the parathyroid glands, pituitary gland, and pancreas.

Thymic carcinoids have also been reported in individuals with MEN1 syndrome.
2. **Neurofibromatosis Type 1 (NF1):** NF1, also known as von Recklinghausen disease, is caused by mutations in the NF1 gene. It primarily leads to the development of neurofibromas, but thymic tumors, including thymomas, have been documented in some individuals with NF1.
3. **22q11.2 Deletion Syndrome (DiGeorge Syndrome):** Individuals with DiGeorge syndrome have a deletion of a segment of chromosome 22. This syndrome is characterized by congenital heart defects, immune system abnormalities, and thymic hypoplasia. Thymic tumors have been reported in rare cases of DiGeorge syndrome.

Clinical Implications:

Understanding the genetic predisposition and familial syndromes associated with thymic tumors has several clinical implications:

1. **Screening and Surveillance:** Individuals with known genetic predispositions or familial syndromes associated with thymic tumors may benefit from regular screening and surveillance to detect thymic malignancies at an early and potentially more treatable stage.
2. **Genetic Counseling:** Genetic counseling is crucial for individuals with hereditary syndromes that increase the risk of thymic tumors. Genetic counselors can provide information about the risk of developing thymic malignancies, discuss genetic testing options, and offer guidance on family planning.
3. **Treatment Considerations:** Thymic tumors that occur in the context of familial syndromes may have unique

clinical characteristics and treatment considerations. A personalized approach to treatment, taking into account the underlying syndrome, is essential.
4. **Research Opportunities:** Investigating the genetic basis of thymic tumors in individuals with a family history or predisposition may provide insights into the underlying mechanisms of tumorigenesis and potentially identify novel therapeutic targets.

Challenges and Future Directions:

Despite the emerging understanding of genetic predisposition and familial syndromes associated with thymic tumors, many questions remain unanswered:

1. **Identification of Specific Genetic Mutations:** While some genetic mutations have been observed in thymic tumors, their functional significance and role in tumorigenesis are not fully elucidated. Further research is needed to identify specific genetic alterations driving these malignancies.
2. **Genetic Risk Assessment:** The establishment of comprehensive genetic risk assessment protocols for thymic tumors, similar to those in place for other cancers, is an area of ongoing development. These protocols would aid in the early identification of individuals at risk.
3. **Therapeutic Implications:** Understanding the genetic underpinnings of thymic tumors may open avenues for targeted therapies tailored to the specific genetic profiles of these malignancies. Clinical trials exploring such therapies are essential.
4. **Multidisciplinary Collaboration:** Addressing the genetic aspects of thymic tumors requires multidisciplinary collaboration between oncologists, geneticists, genetic counselors, and researchers to

integrate genetic testing, counseling, and treatment strategies effectively.

In conclusion, while genetic predisposition and familial syndromes associated with thymic tumors are relatively rare, they represent an important aspect of the broader landscape of thymic malignancies. Continued research and clinical efforts in this field hold promise for improved risk assessment, early detection, and personalized treatment approaches for individuals at higher risk of developing these tumors due to genetic factors.

2.2 Environmental Factors and Carcinogens in Thymic Tumors

Malignant neoplasm of the thymus, while often considered a result of genetic predisposition or sporadic occurrence, can also be influenced by environmental factors and exposure to carcinogens. This section explores the role of environmental factors and carcinogens in the development of thymic tumors, shedding light on potential risk factors and avenues for prevention.

Environmental Factors and Thymic Tumors:

Environmental factors encompass a wide range of external influences that can contribute to the development of cancer. While the exact environmental factors associated with thymic tumors are not as well-established as those for more common cancers, research suggests several potential associations:

1. **Ionizing Radiation:** Exposure to ionizing radiation, such as therapeutic radiation for other cancers or occupational radiation, has been implicated as a risk factor for thymic tumors. High-dose radiation therapy to the chest, especially during childhood or adolescence, may increase the risk of thymic

malignancies. This is of particular concern for survivors of pediatric cancers who received chest irradiation.
2. **Environmental Toxins:** Exposure to environmental toxins and pollutants has been studied in relation to various cancers. While direct evidence linking specific environmental toxins to thymic tumors is limited, the presence of carcinogenic substances in the environment raises questions about potential risks. Research into the impact of environmental toxins on thymic cancer risk is ongoing.
3. **Occupational Exposures:** Certain occupational exposures may pose a risk for thymic tumors. Individuals working in industries involving chemical exposure or hazardous materials may face an elevated risk, although the extent of this risk remains uncertain and is an area of ongoing investigation.
4. **Lifestyle Factors:** Lifestyle choices, such as smoking and dietary habits, can influence cancer risk in general. While there is no direct evidence linking these factors to thymic tumors, maintaining a healthy lifestyle can contribute to overall well-being and may indirectly impact cancer risk.
5. **Geographic Variations:** Some studies have suggested geographic variations in the incidence of thymic tumors. However, these variations may be influenced by a combination of genetic, environmental, and demographic factors, making it challenging to pinpoint specific environmental causes.

Carcinogens and Thymic Tumors:

Carcinogens are substances or agents that have the potential to cause cancer by altering the genetic material within cells or disrupting normal cellular processes. Several carcinogens have been identified or proposed in the context of thymic tumors:

1. **Radiation:** Ionizing radiation, including therapeutic radiation used to treat other cancers, is a known carcinogen. High doses of ionizing radiation to the chest area, particularly during childhood or adolescence, can damage DNA and increase the risk of thymic tumors.
2. **Chemical Carcinogens:** Certain chemicals and industrial compounds have carcinogenic properties and may pose a risk to individuals exposed to them. Research into specific chemical carcinogens linked to thymic tumors is ongoing.
3. **Tobacco Smoke:** Smoking is a well-established risk factor for various cancers, including lung cancer. While there is no direct evidence linking tobacco smoke to thymic tumors, the harmful chemicals in cigarette smoke could potentially contribute to carcinogenesis.
4. **Occupational Exposures:** Occupational exposure to carcinogenic substances, such as asbestos or benzene, has been associated with an increased risk of various cancers. Studies investigating occupational carcinogens and thymic tumors are limited but may provide insights in the future.
5. **Infectious Agents:** Some cancers are caused by infectious agents, such as human papillomavirus (HPV) and hepatitis B and C viruses. There is no strong evidence linking infectious agents to thymic tumors, but ongoing research explores potential associations.

Challenges in Establishing Causation:

Determining a direct cause-and-effect relationship between environmental factors or specific carcinogens and thymic tumors presents several challenges:

1. **Rare Incidence:** Thymic tumors are rare, making it difficult to conduct large-scale epidemiological studies

to establish clear associations with environmental factors.
2. **Latency Period:** Cancer often develops years or even decades after exposure to carcinogens. This latency period makes it challenging to link specific exposures to thymic tumors.
3. **Multiple Factors:** The development of cancer is typically multifactorial, involving a combination of genetic, environmental, and lifestyle factors. Isolating the contribution of a single environmental factor can be complex.
4. **Limited Data:** Data on environmental exposures and thymic tumors are often limited, particularly for rare cancers like those of the thymus. Large-scale, long-term studies are needed to gather more comprehensive data.

Prevention and Risk Reduction:

While the precise environmental causes of thymic tumors remain elusive, individuals can take proactive steps to reduce their overall cancer risk:

1. **Avoiding Smoking:** Since smoking is a known risk factor for various cancers, including lung cancer, abstaining from smoking or seeking smoking cessation support can reduce cancer risk.
2. **Occupational Safety:** Individuals working in industries with potential carcinogen exposure should adhere to safety protocols and use protective equipment as recommended by occupational health guidelines.
3. **Radiation Safety:** Patients undergoing radiation therapy for other medical conditions should discuss potential risks and benefits with their healthcare providers. Pediatric cancer survivors who received chest irradiation should undergo appropriate long-

term monitoring.
4. **Healthy Lifestyle:** Maintaining a healthy lifestyle, including a balanced diet, regular exercise, and stress management, can support overall well-being and potentially reduce cancer risk indirectly.
5. **Environmental Awareness:** Being mindful of environmental factors and advocating for environmental protection measures can contribute to a safer and healthier living environment for all.

In conclusion, while the role of environmental factors and carcinogens in the development of thymic tumors is not fully elucidated, ongoing research seeks to uncover potential associations and mechanisms. Until more conclusive evidence emerges, a holistic approach to cancer prevention and risk reduction, coupled with continued scientific investigation, remains essential in the fight against thymic malignancies and cancer in general.

2.3 Immunological Factors in Thymic Tumors

The intricate interplay between the immune system and cancer is a topic of profound significance in oncology. Thymic tumors, which originate from the thymus, an organ central to the immune system, provide a unique platform for exploring the role of immunological factors in cancer development, progression, and treatment. This section delves into the complex relationship between immunology and thymic tumors, shedding light on the multifaceted interactions that define this realm.

The Thymus: A Nexus of Immune System Education:

The thymus, nestled in the mediastinum behind the sternum, plays a pivotal role in the development and education of T lymphocytes (T cells), a critical component of the adaptive immune system. The thymus serves as a "school" for T cells, where they undergo a rigorous educational process to become mature and functional immune defenders.

Positive and Negative Selection: Thymocytes, the immature precursors of T cells, journey through the thymus, interacting with thymic epithelial cells (TECs) that present self-antigens. This interaction results in a selection process crucial for the immune system's proper functioning:

1. **Positive Selection:** Thymocytes that can bind to self-antigens presented by major histocompatibility complexes (MHC) with moderate affinity receive a "survival signal." These positively selected thymocytes proceed to the next stage of maturation. Positive selection ensures that T cells are capable of recognizing a wide range of antigens.
2. **Negative Selection:** Thymocytes that bind too strongly to self-antigens, indicating a high risk of autoimmunity, undergo apoptosis (cell death) in the cortex of the thymus. Negative selection eliminates autoreactive T cells, preventing them from causing harm to the body's own tissues.

T Cell Receptor Rearrangement: During their journey through the thymus, thymocytes undergo a process called T cell receptor (TCR) rearrangement. This genetic reshuffling results in a diverse array of TCRs, enabling T cells to recognize a vast array of antigens.

T Regulatory (Treg) Cells: The thymus also plays a role in the generation of T regulatory (Treg) cells, a specialized subset of T cells that help maintain immune tolerance and prevent autoimmune reactions. Tregs are essential for controlling immune responses and maintaining self-tolerance.

Immunological Factors in Thymic Tumors:

Understanding the immunological factors at play in thymic tumors requires a multifaceted examination:

Immune Infiltration: Thymic tumors, particularly thymomas, often exhibit immune cell infiltration. Lymphocytes, including T cells and B cells, are commonly found in and around thymic tumors. The presence of these immune cells can have implications for tumor behavior and prognosis.

Tumor Antigenicity: The thymus is a site of immune education, where tolerance to self-antigens is established. However, in cases where tumors arise from the thymus, they may express self-antigens that are not typically encountered in the periphery. This can result in an immune response against the tumor.

Autoimmune Paraneoplastic Syndromes: Thymic tumors are known to be associated with autoimmune paraneoplastic syndromes, in which the immune system mistakenly targets normal tissues in the body. For example, Myasthenia Gravis, a neuromuscular disorder, is commonly linked to thymomas. These syndromes highlight the intricate relationship between thymic tumors and the immune system.

Immunotherapy: Immunotherapy, which harnesses the body's immune system to target and destroy cancer cells, has emerged as a promising approach in cancer treatment. Immune checkpoint inhibitors, such as pembrolizumab and nivolumab, have shown efficacy in the treatment of thymic carcinomas, emphasizing the potential immunogenicity of these tumors.

Challenges and Considerations:

While the immunological factors in thymic tumors hold promise for novel therapeutic approaches, several challenges and considerations exist:

1. **Tumor Heterogeneity:** Thymic tumors are highly heterogeneous, both in terms of histological subtypes and immune microenvironments. Understanding these variations is essential for tailoring immunotherapies to specific tumor types.
2. **Tumor Immune Evasion:** Some thymic tumors can employ mechanisms to evade immune surveillance, such as downregulating MHC molecules or expressing immune checkpoint molecules like PD-L1. These mechanisms can hinder the effectiveness of immunotherapies.
3. **Treatment Timing:** The timing of immunotherapy in the management of thymic tumors is a subject of ongoing research. Determining the optimal treatment sequence, whether as first-line therapy or in combination with other modalities, is essential for maximizing therapeutic benefits.
4. **Autoimmune Complications:** The use of immunotherapy in thymic tumors can sometimes lead to immune-related adverse events, including exacerbation of preexisting autoimmune paraneoplastic syndromes. Managing these complications requires a delicate balance between controlling the tumor and preventing autoimmune reactions.

Future Directions and Potential Breakthroughs:

The study of immunological factors in thymic tumors is a dynamic field with significant potential for breakthroughs:

1. **Biomarkers for Immunotherapy:** Identifying reliable biomarkers that predict immunotherapy response in thymic tumors can help personalize treatment

approaches and improve patient outcomes.
2. **Combination Therapies:** Exploring combination therapies that integrate immunotherapy with other modalities, such as targeted therapy or chemotherapy, may enhance treatment efficacy.
3. **Immune Modulation:** Investigating strategies to modulate the immune microenvironment within thymic tumors, potentially rendering them more responsive to immunotherapies.
4. **Enhanced Understanding:** Gaining a deeper understanding of the mechanisms underlying immune evasion in thymic tumors can inform the development of interventions to counteract these mechanisms.
5. **Immunotherapy in Thymic Carcinomas:** Further research into the use of immunotherapy, particularly immune checkpoint inhibitors, in thymic carcinomas may expand treatment options for patients with these aggressive tumors.

In conclusion, the relationship between immunological factors and thymic tumors is a complex and evolving area of study. The thymus, with its central role in immune education, offers a unique perspective on the interactions between the immune system and cancer. As our understanding of thymic tumors and immunotherapy advances, there is hope for more effective treatments and improved outcomes for individuals facing these rare and challenging malignancies.

2.4 Viral and Infectious Associations in Thymic Tumors

The etiology of thymic tumors is a multifaceted puzzle, and emerging research has raised intriguing questions about the potential role of viral and infectious agents in their development. This section explores the connection between viral infections and thymic tumors, shedding light on the complex interplay between infectious agents and cancer within the thymus.

Viruses and Thymic Tumors:

Viruses have long been associated with the development of various cancers, primarily through their ability to disrupt cellular functions, promote genomic instability, and evade immune surveillance. While the relationship between viral infections and thymic tumors is not as well-established as it is for some other cancers, several viruses have been investigated in this context:

1. Epstein-Barr Virus (EBV): EBV, a member of the herpesvirus family, has been implicated in the development of various lymphomas and epithelial malignancies. Although no direct link has been definitively established between EBV and thymic tumors, sporadic reports have suggested the presence of EBV in thymoma samples. The significance of this association remains an area of ongoing research.

2. Human T-cell Lymphotropic Virus Type 1 (HTLV-1): HTLV-1 is a retrovirus known to cause adult T-cell leukemia/lymphoma (ATLL). ATLL is characterized by the malignant transformation of mature T cells. While HTLV-1 primarily affects mature T cells, its potential involvement in thymic tumors is less understood. Research has explored the possibility of HTLV-1 playing a role in thymic tumor development.

3. Human Immunodeficiency Virus (HIV): HIV, the virus responsible for AIDS, can lead to immunodeficiency and an increased risk of certain cancers, including lymphomas and Kaposi's sarcoma. Although the primary impact of HIV is on mature T cells, its effects on thymic function and the potential for thymic tumors in HIV-infected individuals have been areas of interest.

4. Other Viruses: While the above viruses have garnered attention, research into other viruses potentially associated with thymic tumors is ongoing. Viral infections can trigger inflammation and immune responses that may contribute to tumorigenesis. Investigating the presence of various viruses in thymic tumor tissues is part of this exploration.

Infectious Agents and Autoimmune Paraneoplastic Syndromes:

Thymic tumors are well-known for their association with autoimmune paraneoplastic syndromes, in which the immune system mistakenly targets normal tissues. While viruses may not directly cause thymic tumors, their presence could trigger immune responses that contribute to the development of autoimmune paraneoplastic syndromes. These syndromes, such as Myasthenia Gravis, often co-occur with thymomas and thymic carcinomas.

Research Challenges and Future Directions:

Investigating the role of viruses and infectious agents in thymic tumors presents several challenges:

1. **Rare Nature of Thymic Tumors:** Thymic tumors are relatively rare, making it difficult to conduct large-scale epidemiological studies to establish clear associations with viral infections.
2. **Diversity of Thymic Tumors:** Thymic tumors encompass a spectrum of histological subtypes, each with distinct characteristics. It is essential to consider this diversity when exploring viral associations.
3. **Viral Detection:** Detecting viruses in tumor tissues can be challenging, as their presence may be sporadic or require specialized techniques. False positives and negatives can complicate the interpretation of results.

4. **Tumor Immune Microenvironment:** Understanding the interactions between viruses, the immune microenvironment within thymic tumors, and autoimmune responses is a complex endeavor.
5. **Temporal Relationships:** Establishing the temporal relationship between viral infections, autoimmune responses, and thymic tumor development is challenging due to the prolonged latency period often associated with cancer.

Despite these challenges, ongoing research aims to unravel the intricate connections between viral infections and thymic tumors. Some potential future directions include:

1. **Comprehensive Viral Screening:** Conducting comprehensive viral screening in thymic tumor tissues to identify viral agents and assess their prevalence across different histological subtypes.
2. **Viral Genomic Integration:** Exploring whether viruses can integrate their genetic material into the genomes of thymic tumor cells, potentially contributing to tumorigenesis.
3. **Autoimmune Mechanisms:** Investigating the mechanisms by which viral infections may trigger autoimmune responses within the thymus, potentially leading to the development of thymic tumors.
4. **Immunotherapeutic Approaches:** Exploring immunotherapeutic strategies that target both viral infections and cancer within the thymus, particularly in cases of autoimmune paraneoplastic syndromes.
5. **Preventive Measures:** Assessing whether preventive measures, such as vaccinations against specific viruses, could reduce the risk of thymic tumors in susceptible populations.

Conclusion:

The potential link between viral and infectious agents and thymic tumors adds a layer of complexity to our understanding of the etiology of these rare malignancies. While the evidence is not yet conclusive, ongoing research is shedding light on the interactions between viruses, the immune system, and thymic tumor development. As we continue to uncover the nuances of this relationship, it holds the promise of informing future diagnostic, therapeutic, and preventive approaches for individuals affected by thymic tumors and associated autoimmune paraneoplastic syndromes.

2.5 Hormonal Influences in Thymic Tumors

Thymic tumors, a diverse group of rare malignancies arising from the thymus gland, have been a subject of scientific intrigue due to their unique biology and clinical behavior. While the role of hormones in thymic tumor development and progression is not as extensively studied as in some other cancers, emerging research suggests that hormonal influences may play a part in the complex landscape of these tumors. This section explores the potential connections between hormones and thymic tumors, shedding light on the intricate interplay between endocrine factors and cancer within the thymus.

The Thymus and Hormonal Function:

The thymus, located in the anterior mediastinum behind the sternum, is a central organ of the immune system. Its primary function is the production and education of T lymphocytes (T cells), a vital component of the adaptive immune system. Unlike many other organs in the body, the thymus has a distinct life cycle and undergoes involution, or gradual shrinkage, as individuals age. Thymic involution involves the replacement of functional thymic tissue with fatty tissue.

Hormonal Regulation of the Thymus:

Hormones, the chemical messengers of the endocrine system, exert control over various physiological processes throughout the body. The thymus is not exempt from hormonal regulation, and several hormones are known to influence its development and function:

1. **Thymopoietin:** Thymopoietin, a hormone-like peptide, is secreted by the thymic epithelial cells (TECs) within the thymus. It plays a role in thymocyte differentiation and the maturation of T cells.
2. **Thymulin:** Thymulin, also produced by TECs, is essential for T cell development and the maintenance of immune function within the thymus.
3. **Sex Hormones:** Sex hormones, including estrogen, progesterone, and testosterone, have receptors within the thymus and can modulate its function. These hormones influence thymic development and the production of T cells.

Hormonal Influences in Thymic Tumors:

The connection between hormones and thymic tumors is a subject of ongoing research, and several aspects warrant investigation:

1. Hormone Receptor Expression: Research has shown that thymic tumors, particularly thymomas and thymic carcinomas, can express hormone receptors, including estrogen and progesterone receptors. This suggests that these tumors may respond to hormonal signals, potentially influencing their growth and behavior.

2. Gender Disparities: Thymic tumors exhibit gender disparities, with a higher incidence in males compared to females. This gender bias has sparked interest in the potential role of sex hormones in tumor development. While the precise mechanisms are not fully understood, hormonal influences are considered one of the contributing factors.

3. Immune Modulation: Hormones can influence immune responses, and alterations in hormonal levels may impact the immune microenvironment within thymic tumors. Understanding the interactions between hormones, the immune system, and tumor cells is a complex endeavor.

4. Paraneoplastic Syndromes: Some thymic tumors are associated with paraneoplastic syndromes, such as myasthenia gravis, in which hormones may play a role. The relationship between hormones and the development of paraneoplastic syndromes in the context of thymic tumors requires further exploration.

5. Thymic Carcinomas: Thymic carcinomas, a subset of thymic tumors, are often more aggressive than thymomas. Research into the hormonal influences specific to thymic carcinomas may uncover differences in tumor biology and therapeutic opportunities.

Challenges and Future Directions:

Investigating the role of hormones in thymic tumors presents several challenges:

1. **Heterogeneity of Thymic Tumors:** Thymic tumors encompass a spectrum of histological subtypes, each with distinct characteristics. Understanding the role of hormones may require considering this heterogeneity.
2. **Hormone Receptor Expression:** While hormone receptor expression has been observed in thymic tumors, the functional significance of these receptors and their role in tumorigenesis remain areas of exploration.

3. **Gender Disparities:** The reasons behind gender disparities in thymic tumor incidence are not fully elucidated. Hormonal influences are one potential factor, but additional research is needed.
4. **Immune Interactions:** The interactions between hormones, the immune system, and tumor cells within the thymus are complex and multifaceted. Deciphering these interactions is a challenge.
5. **Treatment Implications:** If hormones are found to play a role in thymic tumor development or progression, it may open avenues for novel therapeutic approaches. However, translating these findings into clinical practice will require rigorous investigation.

Future Directions and Potential Breakthroughs:

Exploration of hormonal influences in thymic tumors is an evolving field with the potential for significant breakthroughs:

1. **Hormonal Targeting:** If hormonal influences are confirmed to be significant, targeting hormone receptors within thymic tumors may become a viable therapeutic strategy.
2. **Gender-Based Approaches:** Tailoring treatment approaches based on gender and hormonal factors may lead to improved outcomes for individuals with thymic tumors.
3. **Immune-Hormone Interactions:** Understanding how hormones modulate immune responses within thymic tumors could inform the development of combination therapies targeting both hormonal and immune factors.
4. **Early Detection:** Identifying hormonal markers associated with thymic tumors may lead to improved early detection methods.

In conclusion, the potential role of hormones in thymic tumors adds complexity to our understanding of these rare malignancies. While the evidence is still emerging, ongoing research into hormonal influences within the thymus holds promise for uncovering novel insights into thymic tumor biology and potential therapeutic interventions.

2.6 Emerging Etiological Research in Thymic Tumors

Thymic tumors, a group of rare malignancies originating in the thymus gland, have long captivated the attention of researchers and clinicians due to their unique characteristics and enigmatic origins. While the etiology of thymic tumors has remained a subject of ongoing investigation, emerging research is shedding new light on potential causes and contributing factors. This section delves into the latest findings and emerging areas of research in the quest to unravel the mysteries surrounding the development of thymic tumors.

1. Genetic and Molecular Profiling:

Advancements in genetic and molecular profiling techniques have revolutionized our understanding of cancer biology, including thymic tumors. Emerging research in this area is uncovering intricate genetic alterations and molecular pathways associated with thymic tumor development:

Genetic Mutations: Recent studies have identified specific genetic mutations in thymic tumors, shedding light on potential drivers of tumorigenesis. These mutations include alterations in genes such as KIT, TP53, HRAS, and EGFR. Investigating the functional significance of these mutations and their roles in tumor progression is an active area of research.

Molecular Subtyping: Thymic tumors exhibit considerable

heterogeneity, making it challenging to develop targeted therapies. Researchers are working on molecular subtyping approaches to categorize these tumors based on their genetic and molecular characteristics. This classification may pave the way for more tailored treatment strategies.

Immune Microenvironment: Understanding the immune microenvironment within thymic tumors is a burgeoning field of research. Immune profiling studies aim to decipher the complex interactions between tumor cells, immune cells, and the tumor microenvironment. These insights could inform immunotherapeutic approaches.

2. Epigenetic Modifications:

Epigenetic modifications, which involve changes in gene expression without alterations in the DNA sequence, have emerged as crucial players in cancer development. In thymic tumors, researchers are exploring epigenetic changes as potential etiological factors:

DNA Methylation: Aberrant DNA methylation patterns have been observed in thymic tumors. Epigenetic alterations can silence tumor-suppressor genes and activate oncogenes, contributing to tumorigenesis. Investigating the epigenetic landscape of thymic tumors may reveal novel therapeutic targets.

Histone Modifications: Changes in histone modifications can influence chromatin structure and gene expression. Emerging research is investigating how histone modifications contribute to the dysregulation of key pathways in thymic tumor development.

3. Immunological Factors:

The intricate relationship between thymic tumors and the immune system is a rapidly evolving field of research. Recent discoveries include:

Tumor-Infiltrating Lymphocytes (TILs): Thymic tumors often contain infiltrates of lymphocytes, but the functional significance of these TILs is not fully understood. Emerging research seeks to delineate the roles of TILs in tumor immunity, progression, and response to therapy.

Immune Checkpoint Inhibitors: Immunotherapy, particularly immune checkpoint inhibitors (ICIs), has shown promise in the treatment of thymic tumors. Recent clinical trials have assessed the efficacy of ICIs, such as pembrolizumab and nivolumab, in thymic carcinomas. Ongoing research explores combination therapies and predictive biomarkers to optimize immunotherapy outcomes.

Autoimmune Paraneoplastic Syndromes: The association between thymic tumors and autoimmune paraneoplastic syndromes, such as myasthenia gravis, is a subject of continued investigation. Researchers are exploring the mechanisms by which these syndromes develop and their potential implications for tumor biology.

4. Viral and Infectious Associations:

While not yet definitively established, research into viral and infectious associations in thymic tumors is gaining momentum:

Epstein-Barr Virus (EBV): Studies have suggested a potential link between EBV and thymic tumors. Ongoing research aims to elucidate the prevalence of EBV in thymic tumor tissues and its role, if any, in tumorigenesis.

Human T-cell Lymphotropic Virus Type 1 (HTLV-1): Investigations into the presence and impact of HTLV-1 in thymic tumors are ongoing, particularly in cases where HTLV-1 infection coexists with other risk factors.

5. Hormonal Influences:

Hormonal influences in thymic tumors, including the expression of hormone receptors and gender disparities in incidence, are subjects of emerging research. Researchers are delving into the potential roles of sex hormones and hormone receptors in tumor biology.

6. Environmental Factors and Carcinogens:

Environmental factors, including exposure to radiation, toxins, and occupational hazards, are under scrutiny for their possible contributions to thymic tumor development. Research is investigating associations between environmental exposures and thymic malignancies, albeit in the context of their rarity.

Challenges and Future Directions:

Despite the promising advancements in etiological research, several challenges persist:

1. **Rare Nature of Thymic Tumors:** Thymic tumors are exceedingly rare, making it difficult to conduct large-scale studies with sufficient statistical power. Collaborative efforts and international registries are essential for aggregating data and advancing research.
2. **Tumor Heterogeneity:** Thymic tumors exhibit significant heterogeneity in terms of histology and clinical behavior. Research must account for this diversity to identify subtype-specific etiological factors.
3. **Multifactorial Etiology:** Thymic tumor development likely involves a complex interplay of genetic, epigenetic, environmental, immunological, and hormonal factors. Dissecting these multifactorial interactions is a formidable challenge.
4. **Biomarker Discovery:** The identification of reliable

biomarkers for early detection, risk assessment, and treatment response prediction remains a priority. Biomarker discovery efforts are ongoing, including the exploration of genetic and epigenetic markers.
5. **Clinical Translation:** Translating research findings into clinically actionable strategies for thymic tumor management is a crucial next step. Targeted therapies, immunotherapies, and precision medicine approaches hold promise but require rigorous evaluation.

Conclusion:

Etiological research in thymic tumors is a dynamic and rapidly evolving field. Recent breakthroughs in genetics, epigenetics, immunology, and virology have provided fresh insights into the complex mechanisms underlying thymic tumor development and progression. As researchers continue to unravel the mysteries surrounding these rare malignancies, the potential for improved diagnostic tools, targeted therapies, and ultimately, better outcomes for individuals with thymic tumors becomes increasingly tangible. Collaborative efforts across disciplines and international borders will be instrumental in advancing our understanding and conquering the challenges posed by thymic tumors.

CHAPTER 3: PATHOGENESIS AND MOLECULAR MECHANISMS

3.1 Oncogenic Drivers in Thymic Carcinogenesis

Thymic carcinomas represent a subset of thymic tumors characterized by their aggressive behavior and challenging clinical management. Understanding the oncogenic drivers behind thymic carcinogenesis is critical for developing targeted therapies and improving patient outcomes. This section delves into the complex landscape of oncogenic drivers in thymic carcinomas, exploring the genetic and molecular alterations that fuel the development and progression of these aggressive malignancies.

Genetic Alterations in Thymic Carcinomas:

Thymic carcinomas are genetically heterogeneous, with multiple genetic alterations contributing to their tumorigenesis. Recent research has revealed several key genetic changes associated with these tumors:

1. **Mutations in TP53:** TP53, a tumor suppressor gene, is frequently mutated in thymic carcinomas. TP53 mutations disrupt the normal regulation of cell cycle progression and DNA repair, leading to genomic

instability and uncontrolled cell growth. These mutations are often associated with more aggressive tumor behavior and poor prognosis.
2. **HRAS Mutations:** Activating mutations in the HRAS gene have been identified in a subset of thymic carcinomas. These mutations lead to constitutive activation of the RAS signaling pathway, promoting cell proliferation and survival. HRAS-mutated thymic carcinomas may be more responsive to targeted therapies directed at the RAS pathway.
3. **EGFR Alterations:** Epidermal growth factor receptor (EGFR) alterations, including mutations and amplifications, have been detected in some thymic carcinomas. EGFR dysregulation can activate downstream signaling pathways, promoting cell growth and survival. Targeted therapies, such as EGFR inhibitors, are being explored as potential treatment options for tumors with EGFR alterations.
4. **KIT Mutations:** Mutations in the KIT gene have also been identified in a subset of thymic carcinomas. KIT mutations can lead to constitutive activation of the KIT receptor tyrosine kinase, driving tumor growth. Targeted therapies that inhibit KIT signaling are being investigated for their efficacy in these tumors.
5. **Other Genetic Changes:** Thymic carcinomas exhibit additional genetic alterations, including mutations in genes such as PIK3CA and BRAF. These mutations can activate signaling pathways involved in cell growth and proliferation.

Molecular Subtyping of Thymic Carcinomas:

Recognizing the genetic and molecular heterogeneity of thymic carcinomas, efforts have been made to classify these tumors into distinct molecular subtypes. This classification helps tailor treatment approaches and predict clinical outcomes:

1. **Squamous Cell Carcinoma (SCC)-Like Subtype:** This subtype is characterized by frequent TP53 mutations, which are often associated with aggressive tumor behavior. SCC-like thymic carcinomas may benefit from therapies targeting TP53-related pathways.
2. **Adenocarcinoma (AC)-Like Subtype:** AC-like thymic carcinomas are often associated with EGFR alterations. Targeting the EGFR pathway with inhibitors such as gefitinib or erlotinib has shown promise in this subtype.
3. **Neuroendocrine-Like Subtype:** This subtype includes tumors with neuroendocrine features and may exhibit KIT mutations. Targeted therapies directed at KIT signaling pathways are being explored for neuroendocrine-like thymic carcinomas.
4. **Other Subtypes:** Thymic carcinomas may exhibit additional genetic alterations or molecular features that do not fit neatly into the above categories. Comprehensive molecular profiling is essential for understanding the unique characteristics of these tumors.

Immunological Factors in Thymic Carcinomas:

In addition to genetic and molecular alterations, thymic carcinomas often have intricate interactions with the immune system. The presence of immune cell infiltrates and the expression of immune checkpoint molecules have important implications for tumor behavior and therapeutic approaches:

1. **Immune Infiltrates:** Thymic carcinomas frequently contain immune cell infiltrates, including lymphocytes and macrophages. These immune cells may influence the tumor microenvironment and potentially respond

to immunotherapies.
2. **PD-L1 Expression:** Programmed death-ligand 1 (PD-L1) expression has been observed in thymic carcinomas. PD-L1 binds to PD-1 receptors on T cells, dampening the immune response. Checkpoint inhibitors targeting PD-1/PD-L1, such as nivolumab and pembrolizumab, have shown efficacy in some thymic carcinomas, particularly those with PD-L1 expression.
3. **Tumor-Infiltrating Lymphocytes (TILs):** The presence of tumor-infiltrating lymphocytes (TILs) is associated with better outcomes in some thymic carcinomas. TILs may reflect an active immune response against the tumor and suggest potential responsiveness to immunotherapies.

Challenges and Future Directions:

Despite the progress made in understanding the oncogenic drivers in thymic carcinomas, several challenges and areas for future research remain:

1. **Tumor Heterogeneity:** Thymic carcinomas are highly heterogeneous, with varying genetic and molecular profiles. Identifying subtype-specific drivers and developing targeted therapies for each subtype is a complex endeavor.
2. **Resistance Mechanisms:** Tumors often develop resistance to targeted therapies over time. Investigating the mechanisms of resistance and developing strategies to overcome it is crucial for improving treatment outcomes.
3. **Predictive Biomarkers:** Identifying predictive biomarkers for response to targeted therapies and immunotherapies is essential for guiding treatment decisions and improving patient selection.

4. **Combination Therapies:** Exploring the potential benefits of combination therapies that target multiple oncogenic pathways or combine targeted therapies with immunotherapies.
5. **Rare Nature of Thymic Carcinomas:** Thymic carcinomas are rare tumors, making it challenging to conduct large clinical trials. Collaborative efforts and international cooperation are vital for advancing research in this field.

Conclusion:

Understanding the oncogenic drivers in thymic carcinomas is a critical step toward developing effective therapies and improving outcomes for patients with these aggressive malignancies. Genetic and molecular profiling, coupled with the classification of tumors into molecular subtypes, is guiding the development of targeted treatments. Additionally, the complex interplay between thymic carcinomas and the immune system is opening doors to immunotherapeutic approaches. As research continues to unravel the intricacies of thymic carcinoma biology, there is hope for more tailored and effective treatments for individuals facing this challenging cancer.

3.2 Alterations in Tumor Suppressor Genes in Thymic Tumors

Tumor suppressor genes play a crucial role in maintaining the normal regulation of cell growth, preventing uncontrolled proliferation, and safeguarding against the development of cancer. In thymic tumors, including thymomas and thymic carcinomas, alterations in tumor suppressor genes are emerging as key drivers of tumorigenesis. This section explores the significance of tumor suppressor gene alterations in thymic tumors, shedding light on their roles in the development and progression of these neoplasms.

Tumor Suppressor Genes and Their Functions:

Tumor suppressor genes are critical guardians of genomic stability and cellular homeostasis. They act as "brakes" on cell division and growth, ensuring that cells do not replicate uncontrollably or evade programmed cell death (apoptosis). Mutations or alterations in these genes can unleash unchecked cell proliferation, contributing to the initiation and progression of cancer. Some well-known tumor suppressor genes include:

1. **TP53 (p53):** Often referred to as the "guardian of the genome," TP53 plays a central role in monitoring DNA integrity. When DNA damage occurs, TP53 activates pathways that either repair the damage or induce apoptosis to eliminate damaged cells. Mutations in TP53 can lead to genomic instability and resistance to apoptosis, fostering tumor development.
2. **RB1 (Retinoblastoma):** The RB1 gene controls the cell cycle by inhibiting the progression from the G1 phase to the S phase. Loss or inactivation of RB1 allows cells to bypass this checkpoint and replicate their DNA, a hallmark of cancer cells.
3. **PTEN (Phosphatase and Tensin Homolog):** PTEN is involved in regulating cell growth and preventing excessive signaling through the PI3K/AKT/mTOR pathway. Loss of PTEN function can lead to uncontrolled cell proliferation and survival.
4. **CDKN2A (p16INK4a):** CDKN2A encodes p16INK4a, a protein that inhibits the cyclin-dependent kinases (CDKs) responsible for driving the cell cycle forward. Inactivation of CDKN2A results in the unimpeded progression of the cell cycle.

Tumor Suppressor Alterations in Thymic Tumors:

Thymic tumors, including both thymomas and thymic carcinomas, exhibit alterations in tumor suppressor genes that contribute to their development and progression:

1. **TP53 Alterations:** TP53 mutations or loss of TP53 function have been identified in a subset of thymic tumors, particularly in thymic carcinomas. TP53 alterations disrupt the DNA damage response and apoptosis pathways, allowing tumor cells to evade cell cycle checkpoints and accumulate genetic mutations.
2. **RB1 Alterations:** Alterations in the RB1 gene are less common but have been reported in thymic carcinomas. Loss of RB1 function can lead to uncontrolled cell cycle progression and increased cell proliferation.
3. **PTEN Alterations:** PTEN alterations, including mutations and deletions, have been observed in thymic tumors. Loss of PTEN function can result in the activation of the PI3K/AKT/mTOR pathway, promoting cell growth and survival.
4. **CDKN2A Alterations:** CDKN2A alterations, such as deletions or inactivating mutations, have been detected in some thymic tumors. Loss of CDKN2A function allows cells to bypass cell cycle regulation, contributing to tumor growth.

Functional Consequences of Tumor Suppressor Alterations:

The alterations in tumor suppressor genes in thymic tumors have functional consequences that drive tumorigenesis:

1. **Uncontrolled Cell Proliferation:** Loss or inactivation of tumor suppressor genes, such as TP53, RB1, and CDKN2A, results in uncontrolled cell proliferation. Tumor cells can replicate rapidly and accumulate, forming a mass within the thymus.
2. **Genomic Instability:** Tumor suppressor gene

alterations can lead to genomic instability, characterized by an increased rate of genetic mutations and chromosomal abnormalities. Genomic instability fuels the genetic diversity seen in thymic tumors, contributing to their heterogeneity.
3. **Resistance to Apoptosis:** Alterations in TP53 and other apoptotic regulators render tumor cells resistant to apoptosis, allowing them to evade programmed cell death even in the presence of DNA damage or other stressors.
4. **Immune Evasion:** Dysregulation of tumor suppressor genes may impact the immune response within thymic tumors. For example, alterations in TP53 can affect the expression of immune-related genes and influence the interactions between tumor cells and immune cells.

Therapeutic Implications:

Understanding the role of tumor suppressor gene alterations in thymic tumors has important therapeutic implications:

1. **Targeted Therapies:** Targeted therapies that aim to restore or mimic the functions of tumor suppressor genes are being explored in various cancers. In the context of thymic tumors, therapies that target specific pathways affected by these alterations may offer therapeutic benefits.
2. **Immunotherapy:** Immunotherapeutic approaches, particularly immune checkpoint inhibitors, have shown promise in treating thymic tumors. Tumor cells with altered tumor suppressor genes may have distinct immunological profiles that make them responsive to immunotherapy.
3. **Combination Therapies:** Combining targeted therapies that address specific alterations in tumor suppressor genes with immunotherapies could represent a

synergistic approach to treating thymic tumors.
4. **Precision Medicine:** As our understanding of the genetic and molecular landscape of thymic tumors advances, precision medicine approaches that tailor treatments to the specific genetic alterations present in each patient's tumor may become more feasible.

Challenges and Future Directions:

While progress has been made in recognizing the significance of tumor suppressor gene alterations in thymic tumors, several challenges and avenues for future research persist:

1. **Heterogeneity:** Thymic tumors are genetically heterogeneous, and not all tumors exhibit alterations in the same tumor suppressor genes. Understanding the diversity of alterations and their functional consequences within different subtypes of thymic tumors is essential.
2. **Resistance Mechanisms:** Tumor cells can develop mechanisms to bypass the effects of targeted therapies or restore the functions of tumor suppressor genes. Investigating these resistance mechanisms is crucial for developing more durable treatment strategies.
3. **Predictive Biomarkers:** Identifying reliable biomarkers that can predict response to targeted therapies or immunotherapies based on tumor suppressor gene alterations is a priority.
4. **Clinical Translation:** Translating laboratory findings on the role of tumor suppressor gene alterations into effective clinical treatments for thymic tumor patients remains a complex and ongoing process.

Conclusion:

Alterations in tumor suppressor genes are pivotal events in the development and progression of thymic tumors, including thymomas and thymic carcinomas. These genetic changes unleash uncontrolled cell proliferation, genomic instability, and resistance to apoptosis, contributing to the aggressive nature of these malignancies. Understanding the functional consequences of tumor suppressor gene alterations is critical for the development of targeted therapies and immunotherapeutic approaches that hold promise for improving outcomes in patients with thymic tumors. As research continues to unravel the complexities of tumor suppressor gene alterations in thymic tumors, the potential for more effective and tailored treatments becomes increasingly tangible.

3.3 Signaling Pathways and Molecular Pathways in Thymic Tumors

Thymic tumors, encompassing both thymomas and thymic carcinomas, are characterized by their diverse histological subtypes and complex biology. An intricate web of signaling pathways and molecular processes contributes to the initiation and progression of these neoplasms. This section explores the key signaling pathways and molecular pathways that play pivotal roles in the pathogenesis of thymic tumors, shedding light on potential therapeutic targets and avenues for further research.

1. Notch Signaling Pathway:

The Notch signaling pathway is a fundamental regulator of cell fate determination and plays a critical role in thymic development and T-cell differentiation. Dysregulation of Notch signaling has been implicated in thymic tumor development:

Normal Function: In thymic development, Notch signaling mediates interactions between thymic epithelial cells (TECs) and developing T cells, influencing T-cell lineage commitment and maturation.

Dysregulation in Thymic Tumors: Aberrant activation of Notch signaling has been observed in thymic tumors, particularly thymomas. Notch signaling can promote cell proliferation, survival, and the development of specific thymoma subtypes.

Therapeutic Target: Targeting Notch signaling components, such as gamma-secretase inhibitors, has shown promise in preclinical models of thymic tumors. Further research is needed to evaluate the clinical efficacy of these therapies.

2. PI3K/AKT/mTOR Pathway:

The phosphoinositide 3-kinase (PI3K)/protein kinase B (AKT)/mammalian target of rapamycin (mTOR) pathway is a key regulator of cell growth, proliferation, and survival. Dysregulation of this pathway is common in cancer, including thymic tumors:

Normal Function: The PI3K/AKT/mTOR pathway transduces signals from growth factors and regulates various cellular processes, including protein synthesis and cell cycle progression.

Dysregulation in Thymic Tumors: Alterations in this pathway, such as PTEN loss or PIK3CA mutations, can lead to aberrant activation of PI3K/AKT/mTOR signaling in thymic tumors. This dysregulation promotes cell growth and survival.

Therapeutic Target: Inhibitors targeting components of the PI3K/AKT/mTOR pathway have been explored as potential therapies for thymic tumors, especially those with pathway alterations.

3. Epidermal Growth Factor Receptor (EGFR) Pathway:

The epidermal growth factor receptor (EGFR) pathway is involved in regulating cell growth, proliferation, and survival. Dysregulation of EGFR signaling has been implicated in various cancers, including thymic tumors:

Normal Function: EGFR is a cell surface receptor that, upon activation by ligands such as epidermal growth factor (EGF), initiates downstream signaling cascades that promote cell growth and survival.

Dysregulation in Thymic Tumors: Alterations in EGFR, including mutations and amplifications, have been observed in thymic tumors, particularly thymic carcinomas. Dysregulated EGFR signaling can drive tumor growth and resistance to apoptosis.

Therapeutic Target: Targeting EGFR with inhibitors like gefitinib and erlotinib has shown promise in specific subtypes of thymic tumors with EGFR alterations.

4. Wnt/β-Catenin Signaling Pathway:

The Wnt/β-catenin signaling pathway plays a critical role in embryonic development and tissue homeostasis. Dysregulation of this pathway has been implicated in cancer, including thymic tumors:

Normal Function: In the absence of Wnt ligands, a destruction complex prevents the accumulation of β-catenin, keeping it at low levels. Upon Wnt ligand binding, the destruction complex is inhibited, allowing β-catenin to accumulate and translocate to the nucleus, where it regulates gene expression.

Dysregulation in Thymic Tumors: Aberrant activation of Wnt/β-catenin signaling has been reported in some thymic tumors, contributing to tumor growth and proliferation.

Therapeutic Target: Targeting components of the Wnt/β-catenin pathway is an area of ongoing research, although clinical applications in thymic tumors are still evolving.

5. DNA Repair Pathways:

Maintenance of genomic integrity is crucial for preventing cancer development. Dysfunctional DNA repair pathways can lead to genetic mutations and chromosomal instability, contributing to tumorigenesis:

Normal Function: Cells employ various DNA repair pathways, including base excision repair (BER), nucleotide excision repair (NER), and homologous recombination (HR), to correct DNA damage.

Dysregulation in Thymic Tumors: Thymic tumors may exhibit alterations in DNA repair genes, such as those involved in HR. These alterations can lead to genomic instability and susceptibility to DNA-damaging agents.

Therapeutic Target: The identification of DNA repair pathway alterations in thymic tumors may guide treatment decisions, as these tumors may be sensitive to DNA-damaging therapies or PARP inhibitors.

6. Immune Signaling Pathways:

The immune system plays a vital role in surveillance and defense against cancer. Dysregulation of immune signaling pathways can enable immune evasion by tumor cells:

Normal Function: Immune signaling pathways, including those involving immune checkpoint molecules like PD-1 and PD-L1, regulate the activation and function of immune cells.

Dysregulation in Thymic Tumors: Some thymic tumors exhibit altered immune signaling pathways, influencing the tumor immune microenvironment. For example, PD-L1 expression has been observed in thymic carcinomas, potentially facilitating immune evasion.

Therapeutic Target: Immune checkpoint inhibitors, such as pembrolizumab and nivolumab, have shown efficacy in treating thymic carcinomas with immune signaling alterations, highlighting the potential for immunotherapeutic approaches.

Challenges and Future Directions:

Despite progress in understanding the signaling and molecular pathways in thymic tumors, challenges and future directions persist:

1. **Heterogeneity:** Thymic tumors are highly heterogeneous, both in terms of histology and molecular alterations. Tailoring treatments to the specific pathway alterations in individual tumors remains a challenge.
2. **Resistance Mechanisms:** Tumor cells can develop resistance to targeted therapies through various mechanisms. Investigating these resistance mechanisms is critical for developing more effective treatments.
3. **Biomarker Discovery:** Identifying reliable biomarkers that predict response to targeted therapies or immunotherapies based on pathway alterations is essential for guiding treatment decisions.
4. **Combination Therapies:** Exploring the potential benefits of combination therapies that target multiple pathways or combine targeted therapies with immunotherapies.
5. **Translational Research:** Translating laboratory findings on pathway dysregulation into effective clinical treatments for thymic tumor patients remains a complex and ongoing process.

Conclusion:

Signaling pathways and molecular pathways play pivotal roles in the initiation and progression of thymic tumors, contributing to their clinical diversity and therapeutic challenges. Advances in our understanding of these pathways are opening doors to targeted therapies and immunotherapeutic approaches that hold promise for improving outcomes in patients with thymic tumors. As research continues to unravel the complexities of pathway dysregulation in thymic tumors, the potential for more effective and personalized treatments becomes increasingly attainable. Collaborative efforts across disciplines and international borders will be instrumental in advancing our understanding and conquering the challenges posed by thymic tumors.

3.4 Immune Microenvironment in Thymic Tumors

The immune microenvironment within thymic tumors, comprising a complex interplay of immune cells, cytokines, and immune checkpoints, plays a crucial role in the initiation, progression, and response to treatment of these neoplasms. Understanding the intricate dynamics of the immune microenvironment in thymic tumors is essential for developing novel therapeutic strategies and optimizing patient outcomes. This section explores the composition and significance of the immune microenvironment in thymic tumors, shedding light on its potential as a therapeutic target.

Composition of the Immune Microenvironment:

The immune microenvironment in thymic tumors is characterized by the presence of various immune cell populations, including:

1. **Tumor-Infiltrating Lymphocytes (TILs):** TILs are lymphocytes that have infiltrated the tumor tissue. They include cytotoxic CD8+ T cells, which have the potential to target and destroy tumor cells, as well as CD4+ T helper cells that modulate the immune response.
2. **T Regulatory Cells (Tregs):** Tregs are a subset of CD4+ T cells with immunosuppressive properties. They play a role in maintaining immune tolerance but can also inhibit anti-tumor immune responses.
3. **Myeloid-Derived Suppressor Cells (MDSCs):** MDSCs are a heterogeneous population of myeloid cells with immunosuppressive functions. They can suppress the activity of T cells and promote immune evasion by tumors.
4. **Macrophages:** Tumor-associated macrophages (TAMs) are immune cells with diverse functions. Some TAMs promote inflammation and anti-tumor immunity (M1 phenotype), while others support tumor growth and immune evasion (M2 phenotype).
5. **Natural Killer (NK) Cells:** NK cells are cytotoxic lymphocytes that can directly target and kill tumor cells. Their presence in the immune microenvironment is associated with better outcomes in some thymic tumors.
6. **Dendritic Cells:** Dendritic cells play a crucial role in antigen presentation and immune activation. Their function in the thymic tumor microenvironment is complex and context-dependent.
7. **B Cells:** B cells can contribute to anti-tumor immunity through antibody production and antigen presentation. Their role in thymic tumors is less well understood compared to other immune cell types.

Cytokines and Chemokines:

Cytokines and chemokines are signaling molecules produced by immune cells and tumor cells within the microenvironment. They regulate immune cell trafficking, activation, and function. In thymic tumors, various cytokines and chemokines influence the immune response:

1. **Interleukins (ILs):** IL-2, IL-4, IL-7, and IL-15 are among the interleukins that can impact T cell proliferation and differentiation within the thymic tumor microenvironment.
2. **Tumor Necrosis Factor (TNF):** TNF-α is a pro-inflammatory cytokine that can promote tumor cell death and inflammation.
3. **Chemokines:** Chemokines, such as CXCL12 and CCL2, are involved in recruiting immune cells to the tumor site and shaping the immune microenvironment.

Immune Checkpoints:

Immune checkpoint molecules are critical regulators of immune responses. They can either activate or inhibit immune cells, and their dysregulation in the immune microenvironment can impact anti-tumor immunity. Key immune checkpoint molecules in thymic tumors include:

1. **Programmed Death-1 (PD-1) and Programmed Death-Ligand 1 (PD-L1):** PD-1 is expressed on T cells, while PD-L1 is expressed on tumor cells and other immune cells. Interaction between PD-1 and PD-L1 can suppress T cell activity, allowing tumor cells to evade immune attack.
2. **Cytotoxic T-Lymphocyte Antigen 4 (CTLA-4):** CTLA-4 is another checkpoint molecule expressed on T cells. It can inhibit T cell activation and may contribute to immune suppression in thymic tumors.

Significance of the Immune Microenvironment in Thymic Tumors:

The immune microenvironment in thymic tumors is a dynamic and multifaceted landscape that can influence disease progression and patient outcomes:

1. **Prognostic Value:** The presence of TILs and favorable immune profiles in the tumor microenvironment has been associated with better prognosis in some thymic tumors. High levels of cytotoxic CD8+ T cells, for example, are indicative of an active anti-tumor immune response.
2. **Immunotherapy Response:** Immunotherapeutic approaches, such as immune checkpoint inhibitors targeting PD-1 and PD-L1, have shown promise in treating thymic tumors. Patients with tumors exhibiting high PD-L1 expression or infiltrating lymphocytes may be more likely to respond to immunotherapy.
3. **Immune Evasion Mechanisms:** Thymic tumors can employ various mechanisms to evade immune surveillance, including the upregulation of immune checkpoint molecules like PD-L1 and the recruitment of immunosuppressive cell populations like Tregs and MDSCs.
4. **Tumor-Associated Inflammation:** Inflammation within the tumor microenvironment can influence disease progression and treatment response. In some cases, chronic inflammation may promote tumor growth and immune evasion.

Therapeutic Strategies Targeting the Immune Microenvironment:

Efforts to target the immune microenvironment in thymic

tumors are a rapidly evolving field of research. Several therapeutic strategies aim to enhance anti-tumor immunity and overcome immune evasion:

1. **Immune Checkpoint Inhibitors:** Immune checkpoint inhibitors (ICIs) that target PD-1, PD-L1, and CTLA-4 have shown promising results in clinical trials for thymic tumors. These agents release the brakes on T cell activity, enabling them to attack tumor cells.
2. **Cytokine Therapies:** Cytokine-based therapies, such as interleukin-2 (IL-2) and interferon-alpha (IFN-α), have been explored to stimulate immune responses in thymic tumors.
3. **Adoptive Cell Therapy:** Adoptive cell therapy (ACT) involves the infusion of ex vivo expanded autologous T cells or engineered T cells into patients. ACT has shown efficacy in various cancers and is being investigated in thymic tumors.
4. **Vaccines:** Therapeutic cancer vaccines aim to stimulate the immune system to recognize and target tumor-specific antigens. Vaccine approaches are being explored in thymic tumors.
5. **Combination Therapies:** Combining immunotherapies with conventional chemotherapy or targeted therapies is a strategy to maximize treatment efficacy. For example, combining ICIs with chemotherapy has shown promise in some thymic tumors.

Challenges and Future Directions:

Despite the promise of immunotherapeutic approaches in thymic tumors, challenges and opportunities for future research exist:

1. **Heterogeneity:** Thymic tumors are highly heterogeneous, and the immune microenvironment

can vary between different histological subtypes. Personalized treatment strategies that consider this heterogeneity are needed.
2. **Resistance Mechanisms:** Some thymic tumors may develop resistance to immunotherapies. Understanding the mechanisms of resistance and developing strategies to overcome them is critical.
3. **Biomarker Discovery:** Identifying reliable biomarkers that predict response to immunotherapies and guide treatment decisions is a priority in thymic tumors.
4. **Combination Therapies:** Exploring the potential benefits of combination therapies that target multiple aspects of the immune microenvironment or combine immunotherapies with other treatment modalities.
5. **Translational Research:** Translating findings from preclinical and clinical studies into effective clinical treatments for thymic tumor patients remains an ongoing challenge.

Conclusion:

The immune microenvironment in thymic tumors plays a central role in disease progression and treatment response. Understanding the composition and dynamics of immune cells, cytokines, chemokines, and immune checkpoints within the tumor microenvironment is critical for developing effective immunotherapies and optimizing patient outcomes. Immunotherapeutic approaches, including immune checkpoint inhibitors, hold promise in thymic tumors, and ongoing research efforts are focused on overcoming challenges and further harnessing the potential of the immune system in the fight against these neoplasms.

3.5 Epigenetic Modifications in Thymic Tumors

Epigenetic modifications are dynamic and reversible changes

to DNA and histones that influence gene expression without altering the underlying DNA sequence. In thymic tumors, including thymomas and thymic carcinomas, aberrant epigenetic alterations play a significant role in tumor initiation, progression, and therapeutic response. This section explores the diverse landscape of epigenetic modifications in thymic tumors, highlighting their impact on gene regulation and the potential for targeted therapies.

1. DNA Methylation:

DNA methylation is one of the most extensively studied epigenetic modifications. It involves the addition of a methyl group to the cytosine base of DNA, typically at CpG dinucleotides, leading to gene silencing. In thymic tumors, DNA methylation patterns are frequently altered:

Promoter Hypermethylation: The hypermethylation of gene promoter regions often results in the silencing of tumor suppressor genes, leading to uncontrolled cell growth. Prominent examples include the hypermethylation of CDKN2A and RASSF1A in thymic tumors.

Global Hypomethylation: In contrast to promoter hypermethylation, global hypomethylation refers to the loss of DNA methylation across the genome. It can lead to genomic instability and the activation of oncogenes.

Therapeutic Implications: DNA demethylating agents, such as 5-azacytidine and decitabine, are being investigated as potential treatments for thymic tumors to reverse aberrant DNA methylation patterns and reactivate silenced tumor suppressor genes.

2. Histone Modifications:

Histone proteins package DNA into chromatin, and post-translational modifications of histones can profoundly affect gene expression. Common histone modifications include acetylation, methylation, phosphorylation, and ubiquitination:

Histone Acetylation: Acetylation of histones is generally associated with transcriptional activation. Aberrant histone deacetylation can lead to the silencing of tumor suppressor genes. Histone deacetylase inhibitors (HDAC inhibitors) have been explored as potential therapies in thymic tumors to reverse this silencing.

Histone Methylation: Histone methylation can have diverse effects on gene expression depending on the specific histone residue and the degree of methylation. For example, trimethylation of histone H3 lysine 4 (H3K4me3) is associated with active transcription, while trimethylation of histone H3 lysine 27 (H3K27me3) is associated with gene repression. Dysregulated histone methylation has been observed in thymic tumors, influencing the expression of key genes.

Histone Phosphorylation and Ubiquitination: Phosphorylation and ubiquitination of histones can affect chromatin structure and gene expression. These modifications are involved in various cellular processes, including DNA repair and cell cycle regulation. Dysregulation of these modifications may contribute to the development and progression of thymic tumors.

Therapeutic Implications: Histone-modifying enzymes, such as HDACs and histone methyltransferases, represent potential therapeutic targets in thymic tumors. Small molecules that target these enzymes are being explored for their ability to restore normal histone modification patterns and gene expression.

3. Non-Coding RNAs:

Non-coding RNAs (ncRNAs) are RNA molecules that do not

encode proteins but have important regulatory functions. Two major classes of ncRNAs involved in epigenetic regulation are microRNAs (miRNAs) and long non-coding RNAs (lncRNAs):

MicroRNAs (miRNAs): MiRNAs are small RNA molecules that can post-transcriptionally regulate gene expression by binding to target messenger RNAs (mRNAs) and promoting their degradation or inhibiting translation. Dysregulation of miRNAs has been implicated in thymic tumors, where they can function as oncogenes or tumor suppressors, impacting key cellular processes such as proliferation, apoptosis, and invasion.

Long Non-Coding RNAs (lncRNAs): LncRNAs are longer ncRNAs that can interact with chromatin, transcription factors, and other epigenetic regulators to influence gene expression. Altered expression of lncRNAs has been associated with thymic tumor development and progression, including the regulation of genes involved in cell cycle control and invasion.

Therapeutic Implications: Harnessing the regulatory potential of ncRNAs is an emerging strategy in cancer therapy. Strategies include developing miRNA mimics or inhibitors to restore normal miRNA levels and targeting oncogenic lncRNAs.

4. Chromatin Remodeling:

Chromatin remodeling complexes are responsible for altering the structure of chromatin, making it more or less accessible to transcription factors and the transcriptional machinery. Dysregulation of chromatin remodeling can impact gene expression:

SWI/SNF Complex: Mutations in genes encoding subunits of the SWI/SNF chromatin remodeling complex, such as ARID1A and SMARCA4, have been identified in thymic tumors. These mutations can disrupt normal chromatin structure and gene regulation.

Therapeutic Implications: Targeting chromatin remodeling complexes is an area of ongoing research in cancer therapy. Small molecules that modulate these complexes are being investigated for their potential to restore normal chromatin structure and gene expression.

5. Telomere Length and Telomerase Activity:

Telomeres are repetitive DNA sequences at the ends of chromosomes that protect against genomic instability. Telomere length and telomerase activity play a role in cellular senescence and proliferation:

Telomere Shortening: Telomeres naturally shorten with each cell division. Critically short telomeres can trigger cellular senescence or apoptosis, limiting tumor growth.

Telomerase Activation: Some thymic tumors activate telomerase, an enzyme that can maintain telomere length, allowing for sustained cell proliferation.

Therapeutic Implications: Targeting telomerase activity is a potential strategy for inhibiting the growth of telomerase-positive thymic tumors. Telomerase inhibitors are under investigation as potential therapies.

Clinical Implications and Future Directions:

The recognition of the profound influence of epigenetic modifications in thymic tumors has opened new avenues for research and therapy. However, several challenges and opportunities for future investigation exist:

1. **Personalized Epigenetic Therapies:** The heterogeneity of thymic tumors, both in terms of histology and epigenetic alterations, necessitates personalized

approaches to epigenetic therapy. Biomarkers that predict response to specific epigenetic interventions are needed.
2. **Combination Therapies:** Combining epigenetic therapies with conventional chemotherapy, targeted therapies, or immunotherapies represents a promising strategy. Understanding the interactions between epigenetic and genetic alterations will be crucial in designing effective combinations.
3. **Resistance Mechanisms:** Tumor cells can develop resistance to epigenetic therapies. Investigating the mechanisms of resistance and developing strategies to overcome them is a priority.
4. **Translational Research:** Translating findings from preclinical studies into clinical treatments for thymic tumor patients remains an ongoing challenge.

In conclusion, epigenetic modifications are integral to the development and progression of thymic tumors. Understanding the intricate regulatory networks governed by DNA methylation, histone modifications, ncRNAs, chromatin remodeling, and telomere maintenance is essential for advancing our knowledge of these neoplasms and developing targeted therapies that can modulate epigenetic alterations to restore normal gene expression and halt tumor growth. The future of thymic tumor treatment lies in unraveling the complexities of epigenetic regulation and translating these discoveries into more effective and personalized therapies for patients.

3.6 Advances in Molecular Diagnostics for Thymic Tumors

Molecular diagnostics have revolutionized the field of oncology by enabling the precise characterization of tumors at the molecular level. In the case of thymic tumors, which encompass a diverse range of histological subtypes and genetic alterations, molecular diagnostics play a crucial role in guiding treatment decisions, predicting prognosis, and advancing our understanding of these rare neoplasms. This section explores the recent advances in molecular diagnostics for thymic tumors, including the identification of key genetic alterations and the development of novel diagnostic techniques.

1. Genetic Alterations in Thymic Tumors:

Thymic tumors exhibit a complex genetic landscape, with different histological subtypes often characterized by distinct genetic alterations. Recent advances in molecular diagnostics have elucidated several key genetic alterations associated with thymic tumors:

a. Tumor Suppressor Genes:

- **TP53 Mutations:** TP53 mutations are frequently observed in thymic carcinomas, where they contribute to genomic instability and resistance to therapy. Molecular testing for TP53 mutations can help predict prognosis and guide treatment decisions.
- **CDKN2A Loss:** Deletion or inactivation of CDKN2A, a tumor suppressor gene, is common in thymic tumors, particularly in thymic carcinomas. CDKN2A loss can lead to uncontrolled cell proliferation.

b. Epigenetic Alterations:

- **DNA Methylation Patterns:** DNA methylation profiles can distinguish between different thymic tumor subtypes. Methylation-based classification may aid in diagnosis and prognosis.
- **Histone Modifications:** Dysregulated histone modifications, including histone acetylation and methylation, have been associated with thymic tumor

development. Molecular assays can assess these modifications to inform treatment strategies.

c. Chromosomal Aberrations:

- **Chromosomal Gains and Losses:** Thymic tumors often exhibit chromosomal gains and losses. Techniques such as fluorescence in situ hybridization (FISH) and comparative genomic hybridization (CGH) can identify these alterations and guide treatment decisions.

2. Molecular Subtyping of Thymic Tumors:

Recent efforts have focused on molecularly subtyping thymic tumors to better understand their biology and predict clinical outcomes. Molecular subtyping takes into account the genetic and epigenetic alterations present in each tumor and can lead to more tailored treatment approaches:

a. Thymoma Subtypes:

- **Type A, AB, B1, B2, and B3 Thymomas:** Each of these thymoma subtypes may exhibit distinct genetic and epigenetic profiles. Molecular subtyping can help refine the classification and prognosis of thymomas.

b. Thymic Carcinoma Subtypes:

- **Squamous Cell Carcinoma-like (SCCL) Thymic Carcinoma:** SCCL thymic carcinomas have a molecular profile resembling squamous cell carcinomas of other organs. Identifying this subtype can influence treatment decisions, as it may respond differently to therapy.

3. Liquid Biopsies:

Liquid biopsies have emerged as a non-invasive method for detecting and monitoring genetic alterations in cancer. They involve analyzing circulating tumor DNA (ctDNA) and other biomarkers in blood samples. While liquid biopsies are more commonly used in other cancers, their application in thymic tumors is an area of ongoing research:

a. ctDNA Analysis: ctDNA analysis can detect genetic mutations, including TP53 mutations and other alterations associated with thymic tumors, in blood samples. This non-invasive approach may facilitate monitoring of treatment response and disease progression.

b. Circulating miRNAs: Circulating miRNAs have been investigated as potential biomarkers for thymic tumors. Specific miRNA profiles may provide diagnostic and prognostic information.

4. Next-Generation Sequencing (NGS):

Next-generation sequencing technologies have revolutionized molecular diagnostics by enabling comprehensive profiling of the entire genome, exome, or targeted gene panels. In thymic tumors, NGS has been instrumental in identifying rare and novel genetic alterations:

a. Comprehensive Genomic Profiling: NGS allows for the simultaneous analysis of multiple genes, providing a comprehensive view of the genetic landscape of thymic tumors. This approach can identify actionable mutations and guide targeted therapies.

b. Identification of Rare Mutations: Thymic tumors are characterized by rare mutations and unique genetic alterations. NGS can detect these alterations, contributing to a deeper understanding of thymic tumor biology.

5. Biomarker Discovery:

Advances in molecular diagnostics have paved the way for the discovery of novel biomarkers that can aid in the diagnosis, prognosis, and treatment of thymic tumors:

a. Predictive Biomarkers: Molecular profiling can identify predictive biomarkers that guide treatment decisions. For example, the presence of specific genetic alterations may indicate responsiveness to targeted therapies.

b. Prognostic Biomarkers: Certain genetic alterations or molecular subtypes may be associated with better or worse prognoses. These biomarkers can help tailor treatment strategies and surveillance.

c. Monitoring Biomarkers: Liquid biopsies and other molecular assays can monitor disease progression and treatment response. Changes in ctDNA levels or genetic alterations can provide early indications of recurrence.

6. Targeted Therapies:

Molecular diagnostics are instrumental in identifying potential targets for precision medicine approaches in thymic tumors:

a. Targeted Therapies: Targeted therapies, such as tyrosine kinase inhibitors (TKIs) or immune checkpoint inhibitors, may be selected based on the presence of specific genetic alterations or biomarkers.

b. Clinical Trials: Molecular profiling can help identify eligible patients for clinical trials investigating novel targeted therapies. These trials aim to improve outcomes for patients with thymic tumors.

7. Integration of Molecular Diagnostics into Clinical Practice:

The integration of molecular diagnostics into clinical practice for thymic tumors is an evolving process:

a. **Multidisciplinary Teams:** A multidisciplinary approach involving oncologists, pathologists, radiologists, and molecular biologists is essential for interpreting and applying molecular diagnostic results.

b. **Clinical Guidelines:** Professional organizations and oncology societies are developing guidelines for the use of molecular diagnostics in thymic tumors, ensuring that these tests are used effectively to inform treatment decisions.

c. **Access to Molecular Testing:** Wider access to molecular testing is essential to ensure that all thymic tumor patients can benefit from personalized treatment strategies.

Challenges and Future Directions:

Despite the promising advances in molecular diagnostics for thymic tumors, several challenges and opportunities for future research exist:

1. **Heterogeneity:** Thymic tumors are highly heterogeneous, and not all genetic alterations are present in every tumor. Tailoring treatment strategies to the specific molecular profile of each tumor is a complex task.
2. **Rare Subtypes:** Rare thymic tumor subtypes pose challenges for molecular diagnostics, as they may have unique genetic alterations that require specialized testing.
3. **Validation and Standardization:** Ensuring the accuracy, reproducibility, and standardization of molecular tests is essential for their clinical utility.
4. **Treatment Resistance:** Some thymic tumors may develop resistance to targeted therapies over time, necessitating ongoing monitoring and adjustment of treatment strategies.

5. **Cost and Accessibility:** The cost and availability of molecular testing can be barriers to its widespread adoption, particularly in resource-limited settings.

In conclusion, recent advances in molecular diagnostics have transformed our understanding of thymic tumors and hold great promise for improving patient care. By unraveling the genetic and epigenetic alterations that underlie these neoplasms, molecular diagnostics enable personalized treatment approaches, early detection of recurrence, and the development of novel targeted therapies. As research in this field continues to evolve, the integration of molecular diagnostics into routine clinical practice will play a pivotal role in enhancing the management and outcomes of patients with thymic tumors.

CHAPTER 4: CLINICAL PRESENTATION AND DIAGNOSIS

4.1 Signs and Symptoms of Thymic Tumors

Thymic tumors, although relatively rare, can present with a spectrum of signs and symptoms that vary depending on the type, size, and location of the tumor. Understanding these clinical manifestations is essential for early diagnosis and prompt management. In this section, we delve into the signs and symptoms associated with thymic tumors, including thymomas and thymic carcinomas, and discuss their impact on patients' overall health.

1. Asymptomatic Presentation:

Thymic tumors are often discovered incidentally during routine imaging studies or medical evaluations for unrelated health concerns. Asymptomatic cases are more common in the early stages, particularly with slow-growing thymomas. In such cases, the tumor may not cause noticeable signs or discomfort, leading to delayed diagnosis.

2. Local Symptoms:

When thymic tumors grow in size or invade nearby structures, they can produce local symptoms, which can include:

a. Chest Pain: Thymic tumors may exert pressure on

surrounding structures within the chest cavity, leading to chest pain or discomfort. The pain is typically dull and may be exacerbated by deep breathing or coughing.

b. Cough: Chronic cough, often accompanied by production of blood-tinged sputum (hemoptysis), can result from irritation of the respiratory passages caused by tumor compression.

c. Dyspnea (Shortness of Breath): Large thymic tumors can compress the lungs or airways, leading to difficulty breathing or shortness of breath, especially during physical exertion.

d. Superior Vena Cava Syndrome: In some cases, thymic tumors can obstruct the superior vena cava, the large vein that carries blood from the upper body to the heart. This can lead to a constellation of symptoms, including swelling of the face, neck, and upper chest, along with dilated veins on the chest and arms.

3. Myasthenia Gravis (MG):

One of the hallmark associations with thymic tumors, particularly thymomas, is the development of myasthenia gravis (MG). MG is an autoimmune neuromuscular disorder characterized by muscle weakness and fatigability. Thymic tumors are often discovered in patients with MG, and the relationship between the two conditions is complex:

a. Muscle Weakness: MG primarily affects skeletal muscles and can manifest as weakness in various muscle groups, including those responsible for eye movements, facial expression, swallowing, and limb movements.

b. Ocular Symptoms: Patients with MG may experience drooping eyelids (ptosis), double vision (diplopia), and difficulty maintaining eye gaze.

c. Bulbar Symptoms: Bulbar symptoms in MG involve

weakness in the muscles responsible for speaking and swallowing, leading to dysarthria (slurred speech) and dysphagia (difficulty swallowing).

d. Respiratory Muscle Weakness: Severe cases of MG can lead to respiratory muscle weakness, necessitating mechanical ventilation. This is a life-threatening complication.

The relationship between thymic tumors and MG is believed to be related to autoimmune processes involving the thymus. Thymomas are more commonly associated with MG than thymic carcinomas. The removal of the thymus (thymectomy) is often recommended in MG patients with thymic tumors, as it can improve MG symptoms.

4. Systemic Symptoms:

In some instances, thymic tumors can produce systemic symptoms that affect the overall health and well-being of the patient. These symptoms may include:

a. Fever: Fever is a non-specific symptom that can result from the body's immune response to the tumor or as a paraneoplastic syndrome (abnormal response to cancer).

b. Weight Loss: Unintentional weight loss can occur in patients with advanced thymic tumors, often due to the tumor's metabolic demands and the production of inflammatory molecules.

c. Fatigue: Fatigue is a common symptom in cancer patients and can result from the tumor's effect on energy metabolism, as well as the psychological and emotional impact of a cancer diagnosis.

d. Night Sweats: Night sweats can be associated with thymic tumors, often as part of a paraneoplastic syndrome. They may be severe and disruptive to sleep.

e. Anemia: Some thymic tumors can cause anemia, leading to symptoms such as weakness, pallor, and fatigue.

f. Endocrine Abnormalities: Thymic tumors can impact hormone production and lead to endocrine abnormalities. For example, they may produce hormones such as ACTH (causing Cushing's syndrome) or insulin-like growth factor (IGF, causing hypoglycemia).

5. Paraneoplastic Syndromes:

Thymic tumors are known for their propensity to trigger paraneoplastic syndromes, which are a group of rare disorders caused by the tumor's production of hormones, cytokines, or autoantibodies. Paraneoplastic syndromes can affect various organs and systems and are often unrelated to the physical presence of the tumor. Examples of paraneoplastic syndromes associated with thymic tumors include:

a. Paraneoplastic Neuromyotonia: This syndrome is characterized by muscle stiffness, twitching, and cramps due to autoantibodies that target voltage-gated potassium channels.

b. Paraneoplastic Pemphigus: This rare autoimmune blistering skin disorder can occur in association with thymic tumors and presents with painful skin and mucous membrane lesions.

c. Paraneoplastic Encephalitis: Thymic tumors can lead to autoimmune encephalitis, which can manifest as cognitive impairment, seizures, and psychiatric symptoms.

d. Hypogammaglobulinemia: Some thymic tumors can result in low levels of immunoglobulins (antibodies), leading to an increased risk of infections.

e. Pure Red Cell Aplasia (PRCA): PRCA is a rare disorder characterized by a shortage of red blood cells due to the production of erythropoietin (EPO) by thymic tumors.

It's important to note that paraneoplastic syndromes can be challenging to diagnose and may require the expertise of multiple specialists, including neurologists, dermatologists, and immunologists, in addition to oncologists.

6. Hormone-Related Symptoms:

Thymic tumors, particularly thymomas, can lead to the overproduction of hormones or hormone-like substances, resulting in specific symptoms:

a. Cushing's Syndrome: Excessive production of adrenocorticotropic hormone (ACTH) by thymic tumors can lead to Cushing's syndrome, characterized by symptoms such as weight gain, central obesity, high blood pressure, and skin changes (purple striae).

b. Hypoglycemia: Some thymic tumors produce insulin-like growth factor (IGF), which can lead to hypoglycemia (low blood sugar) with symptoms like confusion, sweating, and shakiness.

7. Diagnostic Challenges:

Due to the wide variability in signs and symptoms associated with thymic tumors, diagnosis can be challenging. Many of these symptoms overlap with other medical conditions, and patients may not initially seek medical attention for what they perceive as minor complaints. Therefore, a high index of suspicion, thorough medical evaluation, and specialized testing are often necessary to confirm the presence of a thymic tumor.

In conclusion, thymic tumors, including thymomas and thymic carcinomas, can present with a diverse array of signs and symptoms, ranging from asymptomatic findings on imaging to more severe complications such as myasthenia gravis, paraneoplastic syndromes, and hormone-related disturbances. Early recognition of these symptoms and prompt evaluation by healthcare professionals are critical for timely diagnosis and the initiation of appropriate treatment strategies. Given the variability in presentation, a multidisciplinary approach involving oncologists, neurologists, pulmonologists, and other specialists is often necessary to provide comprehensive care to patients with thymic tumors.

4.2 Radiological Imaging Techniques for Thymic Tumors

Radiological imaging plays a pivotal role in the diagnosis, staging, and management of thymic tumors, including thymomas and thymic carcinomas. These rare neoplasms often present with diverse clinical manifestations, making accurate imaging assessment essential for treatment planning and monitoring. In this section, we explore the various radiological imaging techniques used to evaluate thymic tumors, emphasizing their strengths, limitations, and clinical applications.

1. Chest X-Ray (CXR):

Chest X-ray is often the initial imaging modality employed when thymic tumors are suspected. While it provides a quick and cost-effective evaluation of the chest, it has limited sensitivity and specificity for detecting thymic tumors, especially in their early stages. However, chest X-rays may reveal certain indirect signs suggestive of a thymic tumor:

a. Anterior Mediastinal Mass: Thymic tumors typically manifest as anterior mediastinal masses, which may appear as soft tissue densities on chest X-ray.

b. Blunting of the Costophrenic Angle: Thymic tumors, if large, can displace adjacent structures, leading to the blunting of the costophrenic angle, which is visible on X-ray.

While chest X-ray alone may not provide a definitive diagnosis, it often serves as the initial step in the imaging workup and can guide further diagnostic imaging.

2. Computed Tomography (CT):

CT imaging is the cornerstone of radiological evaluation for thymic tumors due to its excellent spatial resolution and ability to provide detailed anatomical information. CT scans are performed with or without intravenous contrast enhancement and offer several advantages:

a. Localization and Size: CT accurately localizes thymic tumors within the anterior mediastinum and precisely measures their size and extent. This information is critical for staging and treatment planning.

b. Tumor Characterization: CT can help differentiate thymic tumors from other mediastinal masses by assessing their density. Thymomas typically have soft tissue density, while thymic carcinomas may demonstrate areas of necrosis or calcification.

c. Lymph Node Assessment: CT can evaluate regional lymph nodes for evidence of metastasis. Enlarged or abnormal lymph nodes may suggest lymphatic spread of the tumor.

d. Invasion of Adjacent Structures: CT can identify invasion of adjacent structures such as the pericardium, pleura, and great vessels, which can influence surgical planning.

e. Assessment of Paraneoplastic Syndromes: CT imaging may reveal findings associated with paraneoplastic syndromes, such as thymic carcinomas causing superior vena cava syndrome.

f. Response Assessment: Following treatment, CT scans are used to assess treatment response and monitor for disease recurrence.

However, it's important to note that CT imaging involves ionizing radiation, and the use of intravenous contrast can be contraindicated in some patients with allergies or renal dysfunction.

3. Magnetic Resonance Imaging (MRI):

MRI is another valuable imaging technique for assessing thymic tumors, especially when a non-ionizing radiation option is preferred or additional soft tissue characterization is needed:

a. Tissue Characterization: MRI provides excellent soft tissue contrast, making it valuable for distinguishing between different thymic tumor histologies and for assessing invasion into adjacent structures.

b. Multi-Parametric Imaging: Advanced MRI techniques, such as diffusion-weighted imaging (DWI) and dynamic contrast-enhanced MRI, can provide additional information about tumor cellularity, vascularity, and tissue perfusion.

c. Evaluation of Myasthenia Gravis: MRI of the chest can be useful in assessing the thymus in patients with myasthenia gravis (MG). It can identify thymic hyperplasia, thymomas, or other thymic abnormalities contributing to MG.

d. Avoidance of Ionizing Radiation: MRI does not involve ionizing radiation, making it a safer option for patients who require repeated imaging or those with radiation sensitivity.

e. Functional Imaging: Techniques like MR spectroscopy can provide metabolic information about thymic tumors.

While MRI is advantageous for certain aspects of thymic tumor assessment, it is less commonly used as a standalone modality in the initial evaluation due to factors like longer scan times and limited availability compared to CT.

4. Positron Emission Tomography-Computed Tomography (PET-CT):

PET-CT combines metabolic information obtained from PET with detailed anatomical imaging from CT, offering a comprehensive assessment of thymic tumors. Key advantages of PET-CT in thymic tumor evaluation include:

a. Metabolic Activity: PET-CT can assess the metabolic activity of thymic tumors by measuring the uptake of a radiotracer, typically fluorodeoxyglucose (FDG). Highly metabolic areas may indicate malignancy.

b. Staging: PET-CT is valuable for staging thymic tumors by detecting distant metastases and regional lymph node involvement.

c. Response Assessment: After treatment, PET-CT is used to evaluate treatment response by assessing changes in metabolic activity within the tumor.

d. Diagnosis of Thymic Carcinomas: Thymic carcinomas often demonstrate increased FDG uptake on PET-CT, which can aid in distinguishing them from thymomas.

e. Assessment of Paraneoplastic Syndromes: PET-CT can detect metabolic changes associated with paraneoplastic syndromes, such as increased FDG uptake in muscles affected by myasthenia gravis.

However, it's important to note that PET-CT has limitations, including false positives related to non-malignant conditions with high metabolic activity and false negatives in tumors with low FDG uptake.

5. Endobronchial Ultrasound (EBUS) and Endoscopic Ultrasound (EUS):

EBUS and EUS are specialized imaging techniques that allow for the assessment of mediastinal lymph nodes and masses through the bronchial or esophageal walls, respectively. These techniques are often used for lymph node staging and biopsy in thymic tumors:

a. Lymph Node Assessment: EBUS and EUS provide access to mediastinal lymph nodes for sampling, aiding in the staging of thymic tumors.

b. Guided Biopsies: EBUS and EUS can guide fine-needle aspiration (FNA) or core biopsies of suspicious mediastinal lesions, facilitating pathological diagnosis.

These techniques are typically performed by interventional pulmonologists or gastroenterologists and are particularly useful in cases where lymph node involvement is suspected.

6. Ultrasonography (US):

Ultrasonography is less commonly used for thymic tumor evaluation due to limited visualization of the mediastinum. However, it may be employed in certain scenarios:

a. Thymus Assessment: Ultrasonography can be used to visualize the thymus itself, particularly in cases of thymic hyperplasia or superficial lesions.

b. Ultrasound-Guided Biopsies: In some cases, ultrasound can guide the biopsy of thymic or adjacent mediastinal lesions when other imaging modalities are not feasible.

7. Angiography:

Angiography is rarely used for thymic tumor evaluation

today, as it has largely been replaced by non-invasive imaging techniques. However, it may be considered in select cases where vascular involvement or embolization is being considered as part of treatment planning.

In conclusion, radiological imaging techniques play a critical role in the diagnosis, staging, and management of thymic tumors. Chest X-ray, CT, MRI, PET-CT, EBUS, EUS, and ultrasonography each offer unique advantages and are selected based on clinical indications and patient-specific factors. The choice of imaging modality is often made in collaboration with a multidisciplinary team, including oncologists, radiologists, and surgeons, to ensure accurate diagnosis and optimal treatment planning for patients with thymic tumors. Advances in imaging technology continue to improve our ability to detect and characterize these rare neoplasms, ultimately leading to better patient outcomes.

4.3 Histopathological Assessment of Thymic Tumors

Histopathological assessment is a cornerstone in the diagnosis and classification of thymic tumors. These rare neoplasms originate from the thymus, an organ located in the mediastinum, and encompass a spectrum of histological subtypes, each with distinct characteristics. Accurate histopathological evaluation is crucial for guiding treatment decisions, determining prognosis, and understanding the biological behavior of thymic tumors. In this section, we delve into the intricacies of histopathological assessment of thymic tumors, exploring the various histological subtypes, grading systems, immunohistochemistry, and molecular testing.

1. Thymic Tumor Histological Subtypes:

Thymic tumors exhibit a wide range of histological subtypes, each with its own unique morphological and cellular features. The World Health Organization (WHO) classification system categorizes thymic tumors into the following primary subtypes:

a. Thymoma: Thymomas are the most common histological subtype of thymic tumors and are characterized by the presence of thymic epithelial cells. They are further subdivided into several histological types based on their morphological features:

i. Type A: Type A thymomas are composed of spindle or oval-shaped epithelial cells and are often associated with a favorable prognosis.

ii. Type AB: Type AB thymomas exhibit a combination of spindle cells (resembling Type A) and round or polygonal cells (resembling Type B1).

iii. Type B1: Type B1 thymomas predominantly consist of round or polygonal epithelial cells with minimal lymphocyte infiltration. They tend to have a good prognosis.

iv. Type B2: Type B2 thymomas feature a predominantly round or polygonal cell population but exhibit more pronounced lymphocyte infiltration than B1 thymomas.

v. Type B3: Type B3 thymomas are characterized by sheets of epithelial cells with minimal lymphocyte infiltration and are associated with a higher risk of recurrence.

b. Thymic Carcinoma: Thymic carcinomas are less common than thymomas but are generally more aggressive. They comprise several histological subtypes:

i. Squamous Cell Carcinoma: This subtype resembles squamous cell carcinomas originating in other organs and consists of layers of squamous epithelial cells.

ii. Mucoepidermoid Carcinoma: Mucoepidermoid carcinomas exhibit a mix of mucin-secreting, squamous, and intermediate epithelial cells.

iii. Adenocarcinoma: Thymic adenocarcinomas resemble glandular structures and often exhibit complex architecture.

iv. Neuroendocrine Carcinoma: Thymic neuroendocrine carcinomas, including small cell and large cell neuroendocrine carcinomas, are characterized by neuroendocrine differentiation.

v. Undifferentiated Carcinoma: This category includes tumors with poorly differentiated or anaplastic features.

2. Grading Systems for Thymic Tumors:

In addition to histological subtyping, grading systems are employed to further stratify thymic tumors based on their histopathological features. The two commonly used grading systems are the Masaoka-Koga staging system and the modified WHO system:

a. Masaoka-Koga Staging System: The Masaoka-Koga staging system is primarily used for thymomas and is based on the extent of tumor invasion and its relationship with adjacent structures within the mediastinum:

i. Stage I: The tumor is encapsulated and confined to the thymus.

ii. Stage II: The tumor invades the thymic capsule.

iii. Stage III: The tumor invades nearby structures, such as the pericardium, great vessels, or lung.

iv. Stage IVA: The tumor invades the pleura or pericardium and can be resected completely.

v. Stage IVB: The tumor invades distant organs or structures beyond the mediastinum.

b. Modified WHO Grading System: The modified WHO grading system applies to both thymomas and thymic carcinomas and considers histological features indicative of tumor aggressiveness:

i. Low Grade: This category includes Type A and AB thymomas and low-grade Type B1 thymomas, reflecting their relatively indolent behavior.

ii. Intermediate Grade: Intermediate-grade thymomas encompass Type B1 thymomas with moderate atypia and Type B2 thymomas.

iii. High Grade: High-grade thymomas comprise Type B3 thymomas and thymic carcinomas, reflecting their potential for aggressive behavior.

Grading systems aid in predicting the clinical behavior of thymic tumors and can guide treatment decisions. Low-grade thymomas tend to have a more favorable prognosis, whereas high-grade thymomas and thymic carcinomas are associated with a higher risk of recurrence and metastasis.

3. Immunohistochemistry (IHC):

Immunohistochemistry plays a pivotal role in the histopathological assessment of thymic tumors by identifying specific protein markers expressed within the tumor tissue. IHC assists in distinguishing between various thymic tumor subtypes, particularly in cases with ambiguous histological features. Key immunohistochemical markers for thymic tumors include:

a. CK5/6: Cytokeratin 5/6 is commonly expressed in thymic squamous cell carcinomas and can aid in their diagnosis.

b. CD5: CD5 is expressed in thymic epithelial cells and is useful for identifying thymomas.

c. CD117 (KIT): CD117 is often expressed in thymic carcinomas, particularly in thymic carcinomas with neuroendocrine features.

d. TdT (Terminal Deoxynucleotidyl Transferase): TdT is expressed in immature T lymphocytes and can help distinguish thymic tumors from lymphomas or other mediastinal malignancies.

e. PAX8: PAX8 positivity may be observed in thymic adenocarcinomas.

f. Chromogranin A and Synaptophysin: These neuroendocrine markers are useful in identifying neuroendocrine differentiation in thymic carcinomas.

g. Ki-67: Ki-67 is a proliferation marker that can help assess the growth rate of thymic tumors. High Ki-67 expression is associated with aggressive behavior.

IHC panels are tailored to the specific diagnostic challenges presented by individual cases. Immunohistochemical staining patterns, in conjunction with histological features, aid in differentiating thymic tumors and confirming their histological subtype.

4. Molecular Testing:

Advancements in molecular testing have provided valuable insights into the genetic alterations underlying thymic tumors. Molecular testing is particularly relevant for thymic carcinomas and some thymomas. Key molecular alterations include:

a. Mutations in TP53: TP53 mutations are commonly observed in thymic carcinomas and are associated with a poor prognosis.

b. Mutations in RAS and EGFR: Activating mutations in genes such as RAS and EGFR may be present in a subset of thymic carcinomas, making them potential targets for therapy.

c. TERT Promoter Mutations: TERT promoter mutations have been identified in some thymic carcinomas and may influence prognosis.

d. NF-κB Pathway Activation: Dysregulation of the NF-κB pathway has been implicated in the pathogenesis of thymic tumors.

e. Immunotherapy Biomarkers: Molecular profiling can help identify potential immunotherapy targets, such as PD-L1 expression and tumor mutational burden (TMB).

Molecular testing is evolving and holds promise for guiding targeted therapy approaches in select cases of thymic tumors. Identifying specific molecular alterations can inform treatment decisions, especially in cases refractory to standard therapies.

5. Frozen Section Analysis:

Intraoperative frozen section analysis is occasionally employed during surgical resection of thymic tumors. This rapid histopathological assessment allows surgeons to make immediate decisions regarding the extent of resection and the need for lymph node dissection. Frozen section analysis is particularly valuable when the nature of the mediastinal mass is uncertain, aiding in intraoperative decision-making.

In conclusion, histopathological assessment plays a pivotal role in the diagnosis, classification, and grading of thymic tumors. Differentiating between thymoma subtypes and identifying histological features of thymic carcinomas is essential for treatment planning and prognostic assessment. Immunohistochemistry and, increasingly, molecular testing provide valuable adjuncts to conventional histopathological evaluation, aiding in accurate diagnosis and potential therapeutic targeting. A multidisciplinary approach involving pathologists, oncologists, and surgeons is crucial to ensure comprehensive assessment and management of patients with thymic tumors, given the diverse nature of these neoplasms and the importance of tailored treatment strategies.

4.4 Biomarkers and Serum Markers in Thymic Tumors

Biomarkers and serum markers play a vital role in the diagnosis, prognosis, and monitoring of thymic tumors, including thymomas and thymic carcinomas. These rare neoplasms often present diagnostic challenges, and the identification of specific molecules in blood or tissue can aid in early detection, treatment decision-making, and assessment of treatment response. In this section, we explore the various biomarkers and serum markers associated with thymic tumors, their clinical significance, and their potential for improving patient care.

1. Serum Markers for Thymic Tumors:

Serum markers are substances measurable in the blood that can provide valuable information about the presence or progression of thymic tumors. Several serum markers are associated with thymic tumors, and their clinical utility varies based on the type and stage of the tumor. Some of the key serum markers include:

a. Carcinoembryonic Antigen (CEA): CEA is a glycoprotein normally produced during fetal development but can be elevated in certain cancers, including thymic carcinomas. Elevated CEA levels in the blood may suggest the presence of a thymic carcinoma. However, CEA is not specific to thymic tumors and can be elevated in various other malignancies and non-cancerous conditions.

b. Alpha-Fetoprotein (AFP): AFP is a protein produced during fetal development, primarily by the fetal liver. Elevated AFP levels can be associated with germ cell tumors and certain liver cancers. While AFP is typically not elevated in thymic tumors, its measurement can help rule out other cancer types.

c. Beta-Human Chorionic Gonadotropin (β-hCG): β-hCG is a hormone produced during pregnancy and can be elevated in certain germ cell tumors, including mediastinal germ cell tumors. Thymic tumors are rarely associated with elevated β-hCG levels, but its measurement can be useful when evaluating mediastinal masses.

d. Neuron-Specific Enolase (NSE): NSE is an enzyme found in neural and neuroendocrine tissues. It can be elevated in thymic carcinomas with neuroendocrine features. Elevated NSE levels may indicate the presence of neuroendocrine differentiation within the tumor.

e. Serum Calcium (Hypercalcemia): Hypercalcemia (elevated serum calcium levels) can occur in some cases of thymic tumors, particularly thymomas. This is often associated with the production of parathyroid hormone-related protein (PTHrP) by the tumor, leading to increased calcium levels in the blood.

f. Serum Immunoglobulins: Some thymic tumors, especially Type B3 thymomas, can lead to abnormalities in immunoglobulin levels, resulting in hypogammaglobulinemia. Low levels of immunoglobulins, particularly IgG, may increase the risk of infections.

g. Paraneoplastic Autoantibodies: Thymic tumors are known to trigger paraneoplastic syndromes, which can involve the production of autoantibodies targeting specific neural or muscle antigens. These autoantibodies are often associated with conditions such as myasthenia gravis (e.g., anti-acetylcholine receptor antibodies) and paraneoplastic pemphigus (e.g., anti-desmoglein 3 antibodies). The detection of these autoantibodies can aid in diagnosing associated paraneoplastic syndromes.

It's important to note that while serum markers can provide valuable diagnostic clues, they are not typically used in isolation for the diagnosis of thymic tumors. They are often considered as part of a comprehensive diagnostic workup, which includes imaging, histopathological assessment, and clinical evaluation.

2. Biomarkers for Thymic Tumors:

Biomarkers are molecular or genetic indicators found within tumor tissue or body fluids that can provide insights into the behavior, prognosis, and treatment options for thymic tumors. Advances in biomarker discovery have opened new avenues for personalized medicine and the development of targeted therapies. Here are some notable biomarkers associated with thymic tumors:

a. Masaoka-Koga Staging System: While not a traditional biomarker, the Masaoka-Koga staging system is a key factor in the assessment of thymic tumors. It categorizes tumors based on the extent of invasion and their relationship with adjacent structures within the mediastinum. Staging provides important prognostic information and guides treatment decisions.

b. Tumor Histology: Histological subtype is a crucial biomarker for thymic tumors. Thymomas are classified into several subtypes (Type A, AB, B1, B2, B3), each with distinct clinical behaviors and prognoses. Thymic carcinomas are categorized based on their histology, such as squamous cell carcinoma or neuroendocrine carcinoma. The histological subtype informs treatment strategies and prognosis.

c. Immunohistochemistry (IHC): Immunohistochemical markers expressed within tumor tissue provide insights into the histological subtype and differentiation of thymic tumors. For example, the expression of markers like CD5 and CK5/6 can help distinguish thymomas from thymic carcinomas and guide treatment decisions.

d. Molecular Alterations: Advancements in molecular testing have identified specific genetic alterations associated with thymic tumors. Notable molecular biomarkers include:

i. TP53 Mutations: TP53 mutations are frequently found in thymic carcinomas and are associated with an aggressive clinical course.

ii. RAS and EGFR Mutations: Activating mutations in genes like RAS and EGFR may be present in thymic carcinomas, suggesting potential targeted therapy options.

iii. TERT Promoter Mutations: TERT promoter mutations have been identified in thymic carcinomas and may influence prognosis.

iv. NF-κB Pathway Activation: Dysregulation of the NF-κB pathway has been implicated in the pathogenesis of thymic tumors.

v. PD-L1 Expression: PD-L1 expression in thymic tumors is of interest as it may guide the use of immunotherapy agents such as checkpoint inhibitors.

vi. Tumor Mutational Burden (TMB): TMB assessment can provide insights into the potential responsiveness of thymic tumors to immunotherapy.

Molecular biomarkers are increasingly important in guiding treatment decisions, particularly in cases where standard therapies have limited efficacy. Targeted therapies and immunotherapies are being explored in clinical trials for thymic tumors based on their molecular profiles.

3. Prognostic Biomarkers: Prognostic biomarkers provide information about the likely course of the disease and patient outcomes. In thymic tumors, several factors are considered as prognostic biomarkers, including:

a. Tumor Stage: The Masaoka-Koga staging system, based on tumor invasion and extent, is a critical prognostic factor.

b. Histological Subtype: The histological subtype of thymic tumors informs prognosis, with Type A thymomas having a more favorable outlook compared to Type B3 thymomas and thymic carcinomas.

c. Complete Resection: The extent of surgical resection and the achievement of complete tumor removal are key prognostic factors. R0 resection (complete resection with negative margins) is associated with better outcomes.

d. Tumor Grade: Higher-grade thymomas and thymic carcinomas tend to have a worse prognosis.

e. Molecular Alterations: Specific genetic mutations, such as TP53 mutations, may indicate a poorer prognosis in thymic carcinomas.

f. Paraneoplastic Syndromes: The presence of paraneoplastic syndromes, such as myasthenia gravis or paraneoplastic pemphigus, can impact prognosis and complicate the clinical course.

g. Age and Performance Status: Patient age and performance status are important prognostic factors, with younger patients and those with better performance status generally having improved outcomes.

The identification and understanding of prognostic biomarkers help clinicians tailor treatment plans and provide patients with more accurate prognostic information, enabling shared decision-making.

4. Monitoring Biomarkers: Biomarkers also play a role in monitoring disease progression and treatment response in patients with thymic tumors. For example:

a. Imaging Biomarkers: Radiological imaging, such as CT or PET-CT, can serve as biomarkers to assess changes in tumor size, metabolic activity, and response to treatment.

b. Tumor Markers: Serial measurements of serum markers like CEA and NSE can be used to monitor tumor progression or recurrence.

c. Immunotherapy Biomarkers: The assessment of PD-L1 expression and TMB may guide the use of immune checkpoint inhibitors and help monitor treatment response.

d. Molecular Alterations: Monitoring changes in molecular biomarkers, such as TP53 mutations or TERT promoter mutations, can provide insights into disease evolution and potential targeted therapy options.

In conclusion, biomarkers and serum markers play a critical role in the diagnosis, prognosis, and management of thymic tumors. These markers provide valuable insights into the histological subtype, genetic alterations, and clinical behavior of thymic tumors, enabling personalized treatment strategies. As our understanding of thymic tumor biology and the utility of biomarkers continues to evolve, they hold the potential to improve patient outcomes through more precise diagnostics and targeted therapies. A multidisciplinary approach, involving oncologists, pathologists, and radiologists, is essential for the comprehensive evaluation and care of patients with thymic tumors.

4.5 Staging and Prognostic Factors in Thymic Tumors

Staging and prognostic factors play a pivotal role in the management and clinical decision-making for thymic tumors, which encompass thymomas and thymic carcinomas. These rare neoplasms originate in the thymus, a vital organ in the mediastinum, and their behavior can vary widely. Accurate staging and assessment of prognostic factors are essential for predicting outcomes, guiding treatment strategies, and offering patients the most appropriate care. In this section, we delve into the staging systems and key prognostic factors associated with thymic tumors, shedding light on their clinical significance and impact on patient management.

1. Staging of Thymic Tumors:

Staging is a systematic process that classifies thymic tumors based on their extent of spread, involvement of nearby structures, and distant metastasis. Accurate staging is crucial for determining the appropriate treatment approach and assessing prognosis. Two primary staging systems are commonly used for thymic tumors: the Masaoka-Koga staging system and the American Joint Committee on Cancer (AJCC) staging system.

a. Masaoka-Koga Staging System:

The Masaoka-Koga staging system is the historic and widely accepted staging system specifically designed for thymomas. It focuses on the extent of local invasion and adjacent structure involvement within the mediastinum. The system consists of the following stages:

i. Stage I: In Stage I, the tumor is encapsulated within the thymus and has not invaded adjacent structures. This is often referred to as a "completely encapsulated" or "encapsulated" thymoma.

ii. Stage II: Stage II tumors have invaded the thymic capsule, but there is no involvement of surrounding organs or tissues outside of the thymus.

iii. Stage III: Stage III is further divided into two sub-stages:

- Stage IIIa: Tumors in Stage IIIa have invaded the pleura or pericardium but can be completely resected.

- Stage IIIb: In Stage IIIb, the tumor invasion extends to nearby structures, such as the great vessels or lung, making complete resection more challenging.

iv. Stage IVA: Stage IVA tumors have invaded the pleura or pericardium but can be completely resected. However, these tumors are larger and may require more extensive surgery.

v. Stage IVB: Stage IVB tumors have invaded distant organs or structures beyond the mediastinum, indicating advanced disease with distant metastasis.

The Masaoka-Koga staging system has been valuable in predicting patient outcomes and guiding treatment decisions for thymomas. Early-stage thymomas (Stage I and II) typically have a more favorable prognosis, while advanced-stage thymomas (Stage III and IV) may require more aggressive treatment approaches.

b. American Joint Committee on Cancer (AJCC) Staging System:

The AJCC staging system is commonly used for many cancer types and provides a standardized approach to staging thymic tumors, including thymic carcinomas. The AJCC staging system takes into account tumor size, extent of local invasion, lymph node involvement, and distant metastasis. The latest edition of the AJCC staging system (8th edition) includes the following stages:

i. Stage I: Stage I thymic tumors are localized, small, and confined to the thymus.

ii. Stage II: Stage II tumors have grown beyond the thymus but remain confined to the mediastinum.

iii. Stage III: Stage III tumors have invaded nearby structures in the mediastinum or have spread to regional lymph nodes.

iv. Stage IV: Stage IV tumors are characterized by distant metastasis to organs or structures outside the mediastinum.

While the AJCC staging system provides a broader framework for staging thymic tumors, it may not fully capture the unique characteristics of thymomas and thymic carcinomas. Therefore, the Masaoka-Koga staging system is often used in conjunction with the AJCC system for thymomas.

2. Prognostic Factors in Thymic Tumors:

Prognostic factors are variables that help predict the likely course of the disease and patient outcomes. Prognostic assessment is essential for tailoring treatment plans and providing patients with accurate prognostic information. Several key prognostic factors are associated with thymic tumors:

a. Histological Subtype: The histological subtype of thymic tumors is a crucial prognostic factor. Thymomas are classified into various subtypes, including Type A, AB, B1, B2, and B3, each with distinct clinical behaviors. Type A and AB thymomas tend to have a more favorable prognosis, while Type B3 thymomas and thymic carcinomas are associated with a higher risk of recurrence and metastasis.

b. Tumor Stage: Tumor stage, as determined by the Masaoka-

Koga or AJCC staging system, is a fundamental prognostic factor. Early-stage thymomas (Stage I and II) are generally associated with better outcomes than advanced-stage tumors (Stage III and IV). Complete resection (R0) of the tumor is associated with improved prognosis.

c. Surgical Resection Margin: The extent of surgical resection and the achievement of clear surgical margins (R0 resection) significantly impact prognosis. Complete tumor removal with negative margins is associated with better outcomes compared to incomplete resection or positive margins.

d. Tumor Grade: Tumor grade reflects the level of cellular atypia and mitotic activity within the tumor tissue. Higher-grade thymomas and thymic carcinomas tend to have a worse prognosis compared to lower-grade tumors.

e. Molecular and Genetic Alterations: Specific molecular and genetic alterations within the tumor tissue can influence prognosis. For instance, TP53 mutations are frequently observed in thymic carcinomas and are associated with an aggressive clinical course. Molecular profiling is increasingly relevant for guiding treatment decisions and assessing prognosis.

f. Paraneoplastic Syndromes: The presence of paraneoplastic syndromes, such as myasthenia gravis or paraneoplastic pemphigus, can impact prognosis and complicate the clinical course of thymic tumors. Effective management of these syndromes is crucial for improving overall outcomes.

g. Age and Performance Status: Patient age and performance status are important prognostic factors. Younger patients and those with better performance status generally have improved outcomes.

h. Response to Treatment: The response of thymic tumors to treatment, including surgery, chemotherapy, radiation therapy, and immunotherapy, can provide valuable prognostic information. Achieving a complete response or favorable response to therapy is associated with better long-term outcomes.

i. Lymph Node Involvement: Lymph node involvement is a key prognostic factor, especially in thymic carcinomas. The presence of regional lymph node metastasis may indicate a more advanced stage and potentially worse prognosis.

j. Distant Metastasis: Distant metastasis, indicating advanced disease, is a significant adverse prognostic factor. The presence of distant metastases, such as in the lungs or other organs, often necessitates more aggressive treatment approaches.

In conclusion, staging and prognostic factors are critical in the management of thymic tumors. Accurate staging allows for the appropriate selection of treatment modalities, including surgery, chemotherapy, radiation therapy, and immunotherapy. Prognostic factors help clinicians estimate patient outcomes and guide therapeutic decisions. The multidisciplinary approach involving oncologists, surgeons, radiologists, and pathologists is crucial for comprehensive staging, prognostic assessment, and individualized care of patients with thymic tumors. Advances in molecular profiling and the ongoing exploration of targeted therapies offer promising avenues for improving the prognosis and treatment options for these rare neoplasms.

4.6 Differential Diagnosis and Common Pitfalls in Thymic Tumors

Thymic tumors, encompassing thymomas and thymic carcinomas, are rare neoplasms that can present with a wide range of clinical and radiological findings. Accurate diagnosis is crucial for determining appropriate treatment strategies and ensuring the best possible outcomes for patients. However, thymic tumors can mimic other mediastinal and thoracic conditions, leading to diagnostic challenges and potential pitfalls. In this section, we explore the differential diagnosis of thymic tumors, common diagnostic pitfalls, and strategies to overcome them.

1. Differential Diagnosis:

Thymic tumors can mimic various mediastinal and thoracic conditions, making it essential to consider a broad differential diagnosis. Here are some conditions that may be included in the differential diagnosis of thymic tumors:

a. Thymic Hyperplasia: Thymic hyperplasia refers to an enlargement of the thymus gland due to various causes, including immune-related conditions or physiological changes in children and young adults. Thymic hyperplasia can present as a mediastinal mass on imaging studies and may be mistaken for a thymic tumor.

b. Lymphoma: Mediastinal lymphomas, such as Hodgkin's lymphoma and non-Hodgkin's lymphoma, can manifest as mediastinal masses and share radiological features with thymic tumors. Distinguishing between lymphoma and thymic tumors is crucial, as their treatment and prognosis differ significantly.

c. Germ Cell Tumors: Mediastinal germ cell tumors, particularly teratomas and seminomas, can occur in the anterior mediastinum, close to the thymus. These tumors may present with similar radiological features to thymic tumors and require distinct diagnostic approaches.

d. Neurogenic Tumors: Neurogenic tumors, including neuroblastomas and ganglioneuromas, can occur in the mediastinum and may resemble thymic tumors on imaging studies. Careful evaluation of clinical and radiological findings is necessary to differentiate these entities.

e. Parathyroid Adenomas: Parathyroid adenomas can occasionally be found in the mediastinum, and their proximity to the thymus can lead to diagnostic confusion, particularly when they cause hypercalcemia.

f. Mediastinal Cysts: Various types of mediastinal cysts, such as bronchogenic cysts, pericardial cysts, and cystic thymomas, can present with cystic masses in the mediastinum. These cysts may share radiological characteristics with thymic tumors.

g. Metastatic Lesions: Metastatic lesions from primary cancers in other organs, such as lung cancer or breast cancer, can involve the mediastinum and mimic thymic tumors. Histopathological examination and immunohistochemistry are often required to differentiate metastatic lesions from primary thymic tumors.

h. Infections and Inflammatory Lesions: Infections (e.g., tuberculosis) and inflammatory lesions (e.g., sarcoidosis) can occasionally present as mediastinal masses, raising suspicion for malignancy. A thorough clinical evaluation, including relevant laboratory tests and imaging findings, can help differentiate these conditions.

i. Vascular Lesions: Vascular lesions like aortic aneurysms or dissections can occasionally appear as mediastinal masses on imaging studies, potentially leading to diagnostic confusion.

j. Benign Thymic Lesions: Besides thymomas and thymic carcinomas, benign thymic lesions such as thymic cysts and thymic lipomas may also be encountered and should be considered in the differential diagnosis.

2. Common Diagnostic Pitfalls:

Navigating the diagnostic challenges associated with thymic tumors requires a comprehensive approach and awareness of common pitfalls. Here are some common diagnostic pitfalls and strategies to address them:

a. Inadequate Tissue Sampling: One of the most significant pitfalls in diagnosing thymic tumors is obtaining inadequate tissue samples during biopsy or surgery. Given the heterogeneity of thymic tumors, small or superficial biopsies may not provide sufficient tissue for accurate diagnosis. Surgeons and pathologists should work collaboratively to ensure adequate sampling, potentially through image-guided core biopsies or surgical resection with meticulous attention to preserving tissue integrity.

b. Misinterpretation of Radiological Findings: Thymic tumors can display various radiological features, including solid masses, cystic components, or calcifications. Misinterpretation of these features may lead to incorrect diagnoses. Radiologists should be experienced in evaluating mediastinal masses and consider thymic tumors within the differential diagnosis while also being aware of the various mimickers.

c. Failure to Recognize Paraneoplastic Syndromes: Thymic tumors are known to trigger paraneoplastic syndromes, such as myasthenia gravis or paraneoplastic pemphigus, which can manifest with neurological or dermatological symptoms. Physicians should be vigilant in recognizing these syndromes, as their presence may provide important diagnostic clues.

d. Overlooking Molecular and Genetic Testing: Advancements in molecular and genetic testing have provided valuable insights into thymic tumors' biology and potential therapeutic targets. Failing to utilize these testing modalities may lead to missed opportunities for targeted therapies in specific cases.

e. Misclassification of Histological Subtypes: Thymic tumors encompass various histological subtypes, and misclassification can occur, particularly in tumors with ambiguous features. Comprehensive histopathological assessment, including immunohistochemistry and molecular testing, should be performed to accurately classify tumors.

f. Underestimating the Importance of Staging: Accurate staging of thymic tumors is critical for treatment planning and prognostic assessment. Underestimating the importance of staging or failing to utilize both the Masaoka-Koga and AJCC staging systems when appropriate may result in suboptimal management.

g. Delayed Diagnosis: Thymic tumors can have a protracted clinical course, and delayed diagnosis can occur when symptoms are attributed to other conditions. A high index of suspicion should be maintained, especially in patients with persistent mediastinal masses or paraneoplastic syndromes.

3. Strategies to Overcome Pitfalls:

Overcoming diagnostic pitfalls in thymic tumors requires a multidisciplinary approach involving clinicians, radiologists, pathologists, and surgeons. Here are strategies to address common pitfalls:

a. Multidisciplinary Collaboration: A multidisciplinary tumor board involving experts from various specialties is invaluable in evaluating complex cases of thymic tumors. Collaboration ensures comprehensive assessment and facilitates accurate diagnosis and treatment planning.

b. Adequate Tissue Sampling: Surgeons should aim for adequate tissue sampling during biopsies or surgical resections. Radiological guidance can assist in targeting the most representative areas for biopsy.

c. Expert Radiological Evaluation: Radiologists experienced in thoracic imaging should evaluate mediastinal masses, considering thymic tumors in the differential diagnosis and recognizing atypical features.

d. Awareness of Paraneoplastic Syndromes: Physicians should be vigilant in recognizing paraneoplastic syndromes associated with thymic tumors, as they may be the initial presentation of underlying malignancy.

e. Molecular and Genetic Testing: Molecular profiling and genetic testing should be considered, especially in cases with ambiguous histology or potential therapeutic implications.

f. Regular Follow-up: Patients with mediastinal masses or concerning symptoms should undergo regular follow-up, even if initial evaluations do not reveal a definitive diagnosis. Ongoing evaluation can lead to timely diagnosis and intervention.

g. Consultation with Thymic Tumor Specialists: In challenging cases, seeking consultation with specialists who focus on thymic tumors can provide valuable insights and guidance.

In conclusion, thymic tumors can present diagnostic challenges due to their rarity and diverse clinical and radiological manifestations. A systematic approach, interdisciplinary collaboration, and awareness of potential pitfalls are essential for achieving accurate diagnoses and optimizing patient care. Advances in imaging, molecular diagnostics, and treatment modalities continue to enhance our ability to differentiate thymic tumors from their mimickers and tailor individualized treatment strategies.

CHAPTER 5: TREATMENT APPROACHES

5.1 Surgical Management of Thymic Tumors

Surgery is the cornerstone of treatment for thymic tumors, encompassing thymomas and thymic carcinomas. The primary goal of surgical intervention is to achieve complete tumor resection while minimizing complications and preserving important mediastinal structures. In this section, we explore the surgical management of thymic tumors, including preoperative evaluation, surgical techniques, postoperative care, and emerging approaches.

1. Preoperative Evaluation:

a. Clinical Assessment: Preoperative evaluation begins with a comprehensive clinical assessment, including a detailed medical history and physical examination. Particular attention should be paid to symptoms such as myasthenia gravis (if present), chest pain, cough, or respiratory distress.

b. Imaging Studies: Radiological imaging plays a pivotal role in assessing the extent and characteristics of thymic tumors. Common imaging modalities include:

i. Chest X-ray: Initial evaluation often includes a chest X-ray to identify the location and size of the mediastinal mass.

ii. Computed Tomography (CT) Scan: CT scans provide detailed information about the tumor's size, location, invasion of adjacent structures, and the presence of lymph node involvement or distant metastasis.

iii. Positron Emission Tomography (PET) Scan: PET scans help evaluate the metabolic activity of thymic tumors and identify potential sites of metastasis.

iv. Magnetic Resonance Imaging (MRI): MRI may be used to assess the tumor's relationship with surrounding structures, especially in cases where vascular involvement is suspected.

c. Pulmonary Function Tests: Pulmonary function tests are essential, particularly in patients with large tumors or those with preexisting pulmonary conditions. These tests help assess lung function and guide surgical planning.

d. Myasthenia Gravis Evaluation: Patients with myasthenia gravis (MG) associated with thymic tumors should have their MG symptoms and disease status evaluated preoperatively. Thymectomy may lead to MG symptom improvement or remission in some cases.

e. Cardiac Evaluation: In cases involving tumors close to the heart or major blood vessels, a cardiac evaluation may be necessary to assess cardiac function and determine the suitability of surgery.

2. Surgical Techniques:

The choice of surgical technique for thymic tumor resection depends on factors such as tumor size, invasiveness, and the extent of disease. The following are common surgical approaches:

a. Transsternal Thymectomy: This traditional approach involves a midline sternotomy incision, providing direct access to the mediastinum. It is suitable for tumors of all sizes and is the preferred approach for complete resection of thymomas and thymic carcinomas. Transsternal thymectomy allows excellent visualization and access to the tumor and surrounding structures.

b. Video-Assisted Thoracoscopic Surgery (VATS): VATS is a minimally invasive surgical approach that involves making small incisions and using a camera and specialized instruments to access and resect the thymic tumor. VATS is suitable for select cases of thymic tumors, particularly when tumors are smaller, confined to the thymus, and not invasive. It offers the advantages of reduced postoperative pain and shorter hospital stays compared to open surgery.

c. Robotic-Assisted Thoracoscopic Surgery: Robotic-assisted surgery, similar to VATS, is a minimally invasive approach that employs robotic instruments controlled by the surgeon. It provides enhanced precision and dexterity, making it suitable for complex cases with tumors near vital structures.

d. Extended Thymectomy: Extended thymectomy involves the removal of not only the thymus but also the surrounding fatty tissue and lymph nodes. This approach is often used in the treatment of myasthenia gravis (MG) and early-stage thymomas. It aims to minimize the risk of tumor recurrence and improve MG outcomes.

e. Radical Resection: For thymic carcinomas with invasion of adjacent structures, radical resection may be required. This extensive surgical approach involves en bloc resection of the tumor and involved structures, such as portions of the pericardium, lung, or great vessels. Radical resection aims to achieve complete tumor clearance and may be followed by reconstruction of the affected structures.

f. Transcervical Thymectomy: This approach is utilized in some cases, especially for smaller thymomas or thymic cysts. It involves a cervical incision for accessing the thymus. Transcervical thymectomy is less invasive but is limited in its ability to access certain tumor locations.

3. Intraoperative Considerations:

a. Frozen Section Analysis: Intraoperative frozen section analysis may be performed during surgery to assess tumor margins and confirm the histological diagnosis. This analysis can guide the extent of resection and the need for lymph node dissection.

b. Preservation of Critical Structures: Surgeons must carefully preserve critical structures such as the phrenic nerves, recurrent laryngeal nerves, great vessels, and pericardium when feasible. Preservation of these structures is vital to minimize postoperative complications.

c. Lymph Node Dissection: Lymph node dissection is performed in select cases to assess and remove lymph nodes in the mediastinum. The extent of lymph node dissection depends on the tumor's stage and invasive potential. It may include the anterior and superior mediastinal nodes.

d. Reconstruction: In cases involving extensive resection of structures like the pericardium or lung, reconstruction may be necessary. Techniques such as pericardial patching or lung parenchymal reconstruction can be employed to restore normal anatomy.

4. Postoperative Care:

Postoperative care is essential to monitor patients for complications, manage pain, and facilitate recovery. Close postoperative monitoring includes:

a. Intensive Care Unit (ICU) Stay: Depending on the surgical approach and the patient's condition, an ICU stay may be necessary initially for close monitoring of vital signs and early detection of potential complications.

b. Pain Management: Adequate pain management is crucial to enhance patient comfort and promote early mobilization. A combination of analgesics and regional anesthesia techniques may be employed.

c. Respiratory Support: Patients should receive respiratory support as needed, which may include chest physiotherapy, incentive spirometry, and oxygen supplementation.

d. Early Ambulation: Early mobilization is encouraged to reduce the risk of postoperative complications, such as deep vein thrombosis and pneumonia.

e. Monitoring for Complications: Postoperative complications can include bleeding, infection, arrhythmias, and respiratory issues. Close monitoring and prompt intervention are critical in managing these complications.

f. MG Management: In patients with MG, postoperative management of MG symptoms may require adjustments to medication dosages. Some patients may experience MG symptom improvement or remission after thymectomy.

5. Emerging Approaches:

Advancements in surgical techniques and perioperative care continue to enhance the management of thymic tumors. Emerging approaches and considerations include:

a. Minimally Invasive Surgery: The use of minimally invasive techniques, such as VATS and robotic-assisted surgery, is expanding, offering patients reduced postoperative pain and shorter hospital stays. These approaches are increasingly utilized for select cases.

b. Enhanced Recovery After Surgery (ERAS): ERAS protocols aim to optimize the perioperative care of patients undergoing surgery. These protocols incorporate strategies such as preoperative nutrition, multimodal pain management, and early ambulation to expedite recovery.

c. Targeted Therapies: In some cases, targeted therapies may be employed before or after surgery, particularly for advanced or recurrent thymic carcinomas. Targeted therapies may include tyrosine kinase inhibitors or immune checkpoint inhibitors.

d. Multidisciplinary Care: The involvement of a multidisciplinary team, including surgeons, oncologists, radiologists, and anesthesiologists, is crucial for comprehensive patient care. Collaboration ensures a tailored approach to treatment and optimization of outcomes.

e. Patient Selection: Patient selection for surgical intervention is a critical consideration. In some cases, especially for advanced or unresectable tumors, neoadjuvant chemotherapy or radiation therapy may be employed to downsize the tumor and improve surgical outcomes.

In conclusion, surgical management plays a pivotal role in the treatment of thymic tumors. The choice of surgical approach depends on factors such as tumor size, invasiveness, and location. Surgeons must balance the goals of achieving complete tumor resection while minimizing complications and preserving critical mediastinal structures. Advances in surgical techniques, perioperative care, and adjuvant therapies continue to evolve, offering patients improved outcomes and quality of life. A multidisciplinary approach, with close collaboration among healthcare providers, is essential for the comprehensive care of patients with thymic tumors.

5.2 Radiation Therapy Strategies for Thymic Tumors

Radiation therapy is an essential component of the multimodal approach to treating thymic tumors, including thymomas and thymic carcinomas. Thymic tumors are relatively rare, and the role of radiation therapy varies depending on factors such as tumor stage, resectability, and patient-specific considerations. In this section, we explore the radiation therapy strategies employed in the management of thymic tumors, including its role in different stages, techniques, and emerging approaches.

1. Role of Radiation Therapy in Thymic Tumors:

The use of radiation therapy in thymic tumors is determined by several factors, including tumor stage, surgical resectability, histological subtype, and patient-specific factors. The primary goals of radiation therapy in thymic tumors are:

a. Adjuvant Therapy: Radiation therapy may be used as adjuvant therapy after surgical resection to reduce the risk of local recurrence. It is typically considered for thymic carcinomas and higher-risk thymomas (e.g., Stage III or IV).

b. Neoadjuvant Therapy: In some cases, radiation therapy may be used before surgery (neoadjuvant therapy) to downsize the tumor, facilitate complete resection, or make technically challenging surgeries more feasible.

c. Definitive Therapy: In unresectable or advanced-stage thymic tumors, radiation therapy may serve as definitive therapy to control tumor growth and manage symptoms.

2. Radiation Therapy Techniques:

Several radiation therapy techniques can be employed in the management of thymic tumors, depending on tumor characteristics and clinical goals:

a. External Beam Radiation Therapy (EBRT): EBRT is the most common radiation therapy modality for thymic tumors. It delivers high-energy X-ray beams externally to target the tumor. EBRT can be administered using various techniques, including intensity-modulated radiation therapy (IMRT) and volumetric-modulated arc therapy (VMAT), which allow for precise dose delivery while sparing nearby normal tissues.

b. Proton Beam Therapy: Proton beam therapy is a specialized form of EBRT that uses protons instead of X-rays to target tumors. Proton therapy offers the advantage of delivering radiation with greater precision, reducing radiation exposure to surrounding healthy tissues. This can be particularly beneficial for tumors located near critical structures in the mediastinum.

c. Stereotactic Body Radiation Therapy (SBRT): SBRT is a highly precise form of radiation therapy that delivers high doses of radiation in a few treatment sessions. It is typically used for small, localized thymic tumors or for palliative treatment of symptomatic metastases.

d. Intraoperative Radiation Therapy (IORT): IORT involves delivering radiation directly to the tumor bed during surgery. It is a technique that may be considered in selected cases, particularly for thymic carcinomas with close or positive surgical margins.

e. 3D Conformal Radiation Therapy: This technique uses three-dimensional imaging to precisely shape radiation beams to match the tumor's size and shape while minimizing exposure to surrounding tissues.

f. Brachytherapy: Brachytherapy involves placing radioactive sources directly within or near the tumor. It is not commonly used for thymic tumors but may be considered in specific situations.

3. Radiation Therapy in Different Stages:

The use of radiation therapy in thymic tumors varies depending on the tumor's stage and resectability:

a. Early-Stage Thymomas (Stage I and II): In early-stage thymomas that are completely resected with clear margins, adjuvant radiation therapy is generally not recommended. These patients have a relatively low risk of local recurrence, and radiation therapy is typically reserved for cases with adverse pathological features.

b. Advanced-Stage Thymomas (Stage III and IV): For advanced-stage thymomas (Stage III and IV) or thymic carcinomas, adjuvant radiation therapy is often considered after surgical resection. It helps reduce the risk of local recurrence. In cases where complete resection is not achievable, definitive radiation therapy may be considered.

c. Unresectable or Inoperable Tumors: In cases where surgery is not an option due to the tumor's size, location, or patient comorbidities, radiation therapy serves as definitive treatment to control tumor growth and manage symptoms.

d. Neoadjuvant Therapy: Neoadjuvant radiation therapy may be employed to shrink the tumor before surgery, making it more resectable. This approach is considered in select cases where surgical resection is the primary treatment goal.

e. Palliative Radiation Therapy: Palliative radiation therapy may be indicated for patients with advanced thymic tumors who have symptomatic metastases or locally advanced disease causing significant symptoms. It aims to alleviate pain and improve quality of life.

4. Radiation Dose and Fractionation:

The radiation dose and fractionation schedule for thymic tumors are determined based on the specific clinical scenario and treatment goals. Common approaches include:

a. Adjuvant Radiation Therapy: In adjuvant settings after complete resection, radiation therapy typically involves moderate doses delivered over several weeks (e.g., 45-50 Gy in 1.8-2 Gy fractions). This approach aims to minimize the risk of local recurrence.

b. Definitive Radiation Therapy: For unresectable or inoperable tumors, definitive radiation therapy may involve higher doses (e.g., 60-70 Gy) delivered over a shorter period, often using hypofractionation schedules.

c. Neoadjuvant Radiation Therapy: Neoadjuvant radiation therapy doses are adjusted based on the tumor's response and surgical planning. The goal is to reduce tumor size and improve resectability.

5. Emerging Approaches:

Advancements in radiation therapy for thymic tumors continue to evolve, offering opportunities for improved treatment outcomes and reduced side effects:

a. Proton Beam Therapy: Proton therapy is increasingly used for thymic tumors, particularly in cases where precise dose delivery and sparing of critical structures are paramount. It offers the potential for reduced radiation-related toxicity.

b. Immunotherapy and Radiation: The combination of radiation therapy with immunotherapy, such as immune checkpoint inhibitors, is an area of active research in thymic tumors. This approach aims to enhance the tumor's response to radiation and promote antitumor immune responses.

c. Targeted Radiopharmaceuticals: Emerging targeted

radiopharmaceuticals, such as peptide receptor radionuclide therapy (PRRT), may have a role in the treatment of metastatic thymic tumors by delivering radiation directly to tumor cells expressing specific receptors.

d. Adaptive Radiation Therapy (ART): ART involves modifying the radiation treatment plan based on changes in tumor size, shape, or position during the course of treatment. It ensures that radiation is delivered precisely to the tumor and minimizes exposure to surrounding healthy tissues.

e. Personalized Treatment: Advances in radiomics and molecular profiling may enable the development of personalized radiation therapy plans tailored to an individual patient's tumor characteristics and biology.

In conclusion, radiation therapy is a crucial component of the multimodal approach to treating thymic tumors. Its role varies depending on the tumor's stage, resectability, and clinical goals. With advancements in radiation techniques, dose delivery, and combination therapies, radiation therapy continues to evolve as a valuable tool in the management of thymic tumors. A multidisciplinary approach involving radiation oncologists, thoracic surgeons, medical oncologists, and other specialists is essential to optimize treatment strategies and improve outcomes for patients with thymic tumors.

5.3 Systemic Therapies: Chemotherapy and Targeted Agents for Thymic Tumors

The management of thymic tumors, including thymomas and thymic carcinomas, often involves systemic therapies in addition to surgery and radiation therapy. Chemotherapy and targeted agents play essential roles in treating thymic tumors, especially in advanced stages, recurrent disease, or when complete surgical resection is not achievable. In this section, we explore the use of systemic therapies, including chemotherapy and targeted agents, in the treatment of thymic tumors.

1. Chemotherapy for Thymic Tumors:

a. Indications for Chemotherapy:

- **Advanced Stage:** Chemotherapy is commonly used as the first-line treatment for advanced-stage thymic tumors (Stage III and IV) that are unresectable or have metastasized.
- **Neoadjuvant Therapy:** In some cases, neoadjuvant chemotherapy may be employed to shrink tumors before surgery, improving resectability.
- **Adjuvant Therapy:** Chemotherapy may be considered as adjuvant therapy after surgical resection, particularly for high-risk thymic carcinomas or thymomas with adverse features.
- **Recurrence:** For recurrent thymic tumors, chemotherapy can be utilized to control disease progression and manage symptoms.

b. Chemotherapeutic Agents:

- **Platinum-Based Regimens:** Platinum-based chemotherapy regimens, such as cisplatin or carboplatin in combination with other agents, are commonly used for thymic tumors. These regimens may include drugs like etoposide, doxorubicin, paclitaxel, or cyclophosphamide.
- **Single-Agent Chemotherapy:** In certain cases, single-agent chemotherapy with drugs like cisplatin or paclitaxel may be considered, especially for patients with comorbidities or when combination therapy is not tolerated.

- **Immunosuppressive Agents:** Thymic tumors are associated with autoimmune conditions like myasthenia gravis (MG). Immunosuppressive agents such as corticosteroids and azathioprine may be used to manage MG symptoms, sometimes in combination with chemotherapy.

c. Chemotherapy Response and Monitoring:

- **Response Assessment:** Tumor response to chemotherapy is typically assessed using imaging studies, such as CT scans or PET-CT scans. Response is categorized as complete response (CR), partial response (PR), stable disease (SD), or progressive disease (PD).
- **MG Improvement:** In patients with MG associated with thymic tumors, improvement in MG symptoms, including muscle weakness and fatigue, may be an indicator of chemotherapy response.

2. Targeted Agents for Thymic Tumors:

a. Role of Targeted Therapy:

- **Emerging Approach:** Targeted therapy is an emerging approach in the treatment of thymic tumors, with ongoing research into identifying actionable molecular targets.
- **Potential for Personalized Treatment:** Molecular profiling of thymic tumors may reveal specific genetic alterations that can be targeted with tailored therapies.

b. Targeted Agents Under Investigation:

- **EGFR Inhibitors:** Epidermal growth factor receptor (EGFR) inhibitors, such as erlotinib and gefitinib, have shown promise in some cases of thymic tumors with EGFR mutations.

- **VEGF Inhibitors:** Vascular endothelial growth factor (VEGF) inhibitors like bevacizumab have been investigated in combination with chemotherapy for thymic tumors.
- **mTOR Inhibitors:** Mammalian target of rapamycin (mTOR) inhibitors like everolimus have been studied in thymic carcinomas.
- **Immunotherapy:** Immune checkpoint inhibitors, such as pembrolizumab and nivolumab, have shown activity in thymic carcinomas with high PD-L1 expression.
- **PARP Inhibitors:** Poly(ADP-ribose) polymerase (PARP) inhibitors are being explored in thymic tumors with DNA repair deficiencies.

c. Molecular Profiling: Molecular profiling of thymic tumors is becoming increasingly important in identifying potential targets for targeted therapy. Techniques such as next-generation sequencing (NGS) can reveal genetic alterations that may guide treatment decisions.

3. Combination Therapies:

- **Combining Chemotherapy and Targeted Therapy:** Some clinical trials are investigating the combination of chemotherapy with targeted agents to maximize treatment efficacy. This approach aims to leverage the cytotoxic effects of chemotherapy alongside the targeted inhibition of specific molecular pathways.

4. Immune Checkpoint Inhibitors:

a. Role in Thymic Tumors:

- **Immunotherapy Advances:** Immune checkpoint inhibitors, such as pembrolizumab and nivolumab, have shown significant promise in the treatment of advanced thymic carcinomas.

- **PD-L1 Expression:** These agents are particularly effective in tumors with high programmed death-ligand 1 (PD-L1) expression.

b. Clinical Trials: Clinical trials are ongoing to explore the efficacy and safety of immune checkpoint inhibitors in thymic tumors, including their use as monotherapy or in combination with other agents.

5. Adverse Effects and Management:

a. Chemotherapy Side Effects: Chemotherapy can cause various side effects, including nausea, vomiting, fatigue, hair loss, hematological abnormalities, and neuropathy. Supportive care measures, such as antiemetics and growth factor support, can help manage these side effects.

b. Targeted Therapy Side Effects: Targeted therapy may also have side effects, which can vary depending on the specific agent used. Common side effects include skin rash, diarrhea, hypertension, and proteinuria. Management typically involves dose adjustments and symptomatic treatment.

c. Immune Checkpoint Inhibitor Side Effects: Immune-related adverse events (irAEs) can occur with immune checkpoint inhibitors and may affect various organ systems. These can include skin rashes, colitis, pneumonitis, and endocrine abnormalities. Prompt recognition and management of irAEs are crucial.

6. Ongoing Research and Future Directions:

a. Biomarkers: The identification of reliable biomarkers to predict treatment response and guide therapy selection in thymic tumors is an active area of research. Biomarkers may include molecular alterations, PD-L1 expression, and others.

b. Combination Therapies: Investigating the potential

benefits of combining chemotherapy, targeted therapy, and immunotherapy to improve treatment outcomes and response rates.

c. Personalized Treatment: Advancements in molecular profiling and targeted therapies are paving the way for personalized treatment approaches tailored to the unique genetic characteristics of thymic tumors.

d. Clinical Trials: Participation in clinical trials is encouraged for patients with thymic tumors, as it offers access to cutting-edge therapies and contributes to ongoing research efforts to improve treatment options.

In conclusion, systemic therapies, including chemotherapy, targeted agents, and immunotherapy, have become integral components of the treatment approach for thymic tumors. These therapies are used in various clinical scenarios, including advanced stages, recurrent disease, and cases where complete surgical resection is not achievable. Ongoing research into biomarkers, combination therapies, and personalized treatment strategies holds promise for further improving the outcomes of patients with thymic tumors. A multidisciplinary approach involving medical oncologists, radiation oncologists, and thoracic surgeons is essential to optimize treatment plans and provide comprehensive care for individuals with thymic tumors.

5.4 Immunotherapy in Thymic Carcinomas

Immunotherapy has emerged as a promising treatment modality for a variety of cancers, and thymic carcinomas are no exception. Thymic carcinomas are relatively rare and aggressive tumors that originate from the thymic epithelial cells, and they often present at advanced stages with limited treatment options. In recent years, immune checkpoint inhibitors, a form of immunotherapy, have shown significant potential in the management of thymic carcinomas. This section explores the role of immunotherapy in the treatment of thymic carcinomas, including the mechanisms of action, clinical trials, challenges, and future directions.

1. Understanding Immunotherapy and Immune Checkpoint Inhibitors:

a. Mechanisms of Action:

- **Immune Checkpoints:** The immune system has built-in "checkpoints" that regulate immune responses to prevent excessive activation, which could lead to autoimmune reactions. Immune checkpoint proteins, such as programmed death-1 (PD-1) and cytotoxic T-lymphocyte-associated protein 4 (CTLA-4), play a crucial role in regulating these responses.
- **Immune Escape:** Tumor cells can exploit these immune checkpoints to evade the immune system by inhibiting the activation of T cells and avoiding destruction.
- **Immune Checkpoint Inhibitors (ICIs):** ICIs are drugs that block the interaction between immune checkpoint proteins (e.g., PD-1/PD-L1 or CTLA-4) and their ligands on tumor cells, reviving the immune response against cancer cells.

b. PD-1/PD-L1 Inhibitors:

- **PD-1 and PD-L1:** The PD-1 receptor on T cells interacts with its ligand, PD-L1, which is often overexpressed on tumor cells. This interaction suppresses T cell activity, allowing tumor cells to escape immune surveillance.
- **Inhibitors:** PD-1 inhibitors (e.g., pembrolizumab and nivolumab) block the PD-1/PD-L1 interaction, unleashing the immune system to target and attack

tumor cells.

2. Immunotherapy in Thymic Carcinomas:

a. Rationale for Immunotherapy:

- **High PD-L1 Expression:** Thymic carcinomas have been found to frequently express PD-L1, making them potential candidates for PD-1/PD-L1 inhibitor therapy.
- **Limited Treatment Options:** Thymic carcinomas often present at advanced stages with limited effective treatment options. Immunotherapy offers a novel approach to address these challenging cases.

b. Clinical Trials and Evidence:

- **Clinical Trials:** Several clinical trials have investigated the efficacy of PD-1/PD-L1 inhibitors in thymic carcinomas.
- **Key Studies:** Notable studies include the phase II trials of pembrolizumab and nivolumab, which demonstrated significant antitumor activity in patients with advanced thymic carcinomas. These trials showed durable responses and manageable safety profiles.

c. Clinical Responses:

- **Objective Responses:** Immunotherapy has led to objective responses in a subset of patients with thymic carcinomas, including partial and complete responses.
- **Duration of Response:** Responses to immunotherapy have been reported to be durable, with some patients experiencing prolonged periods of disease control.

3. Challenges and Considerations:

a. Response Heterogeneity:

- **Patient Variation:** Responses to immunotherapy in thymic carcinomas can vary widely among patients, and not all individuals benefit equally.
- **Biomarkers:** Biomarkers to predict which patients are most likely to respond to immunotherapy in thymic carcinomas are still being explored. PD-L1 expression and tumor mutational burden (TMB) are potential indicators but are not consistently predictive.

b. Resistance Mechanisms:

- **Primary and Acquired Resistance:** Some patients may have primary resistance to immunotherapy, while others may develop acquired resistance over time.
- **Resistance Mechanisms:** Resistance mechanisms may include alterations in the tumor microenvironment, genetic mutations, and other immune escape mechanisms.

c. Combination Therapies:

- **Emerging Approaches:** Combining immunotherapy with other treatment modalities, such as chemotherapy or targeted therapy, is an area of active research. Combinations aim to enhance treatment responses and overcome resistance mechanisms.
- **Clinical Trials:** Clinical trials are investigating various combination therapies in thymic carcinomas to improve outcomes.

d. Management of Immune-Related Adverse Events (irAEs):

- **irAEs:** Immunotherapy can lead to immune-related adverse events (irAEs) affecting various organ systems, including the skin, gastrointestinal tract, lungs, and endocrine glands.
- **Prompt Recognition:** Prompt recognition and

management of irAEs are essential to minimize complications and maintain patient safety.

4. Future Directions:

a. Biomarker Discovery:

- **Identification of Predictive Biomarkers:** Continued research is needed to identify reliable biomarkers that can predict responses to immunotherapy in thymic carcinomas. This will help tailor treatment to the patients most likely to benefit.

b. Combination Strategies:

- **Optimizing Combinations:** Further investigation into the optimal combinations of immunotherapy with other treatments, such as chemotherapy or targeted agents, to improve response rates and durability.

c. Understanding Resistance: A deeper understanding of the mechanisms underlying resistance to immunotherapy in thymic carcinomas is crucial to develop strategies to overcome resistance and enhance treatment outcomes.

d. Personalized Approaches: Advancements in molecular profiling may lead to personalized treatment approaches, where therapy is tailored to the specific genetic alterations and immune characteristics of each patient's tumor.

e. Expanded Clinical Trials: Expanding the number of clinical trials for thymic carcinomas will provide more treatment options and generate valuable data to guide future management strategies.

5. Conclusion:

Immunotherapy, particularly PD-1/PD-L1 inhibitors, has shown promising results in the treatment of thymic carcinomas, a subset of thymic tumors characterized by their aggressiveness and limited treatment options. While challenges such as response heterogeneity and resistance mechanisms exist, ongoing research efforts are focused on optimizing treatment strategies, identifying predictive biomarkers, and exploring combination therapies. The potential for durable responses and improved outcomes makes immunotherapy a valuable addition to the therapeutic armamentarium for thymic carcinomas, offering hope for patients facing this challenging disease. A multidisciplinary approach, including collaboration between oncologists, immunologists, and researchers, is essential to advancing the field of immunotherapy in thymic carcinomas and improving patient care.

5.5 Multidisciplinary Approach to Patient Care in Thymic Tumors

The management of thymic tumors, encompassing thymomas and thymic carcinomas, is a complex and multifaceted process that often necessitates a multidisciplinary approach to provide comprehensive care. These rare malignancies, originating in the thymus gland located in the mediastinum, can present unique challenges in diagnosis, treatment planning, and follow-up care. This section explores the crucial role of a multidisciplinary healthcare team in addressing the diverse aspects of patient care in thymic tumors, emphasizing collaboration among specialists from various medical disciplines.

1. Thymic Tumors:

a. Rarity and Complexity: Thymic tumors are rare, accounting for only a small percentage of mediastinal neoplasms. Their rarity and diverse clinical presentations contribute to their complexity in diagnosis and treatment.

b. Histological Variability: Thymic tumors exhibit a wide range of histological subtypes, from indolent thymomas to aggressive thymic carcinomas, each requiring tailored management approaches.

2. The Multidisciplinary Team:

a. Core Team Members:

- **Thoracic Surgeons:** Specialize in surgical interventions, including thymectomy and tumor resection.
- **Medical Oncologists:** Administer systemic therapies such as chemotherapy, targeted agents, and immunotherapy.
- **Radiation Oncologists:** Plan and deliver radiation therapy when indicated.
- **Pathologists:** Provide histological and molecular analysis of tumor samples.
- **Radiologists:** Interpret imaging studies and assist in staging and treatment planning.
- **Pulmonologists:** Address respiratory issues and provide preoperative and postoperative care.
- **Neurologists:** Manage neurological conditions, particularly myasthenia gravis (MG) associated with thymic tumors.
- **Endocrinologists:** Address endocrine disorders and hormonal imbalances.
- **Supportive Care Specialists:** Include nurses, nutritionists, and palliative care providers who enhance the overall quality of patient care.

b. Multidisciplinary Tumor Board:

- **Role:** A central component of the multidisciplinary

approach is the tumor board—a forum where specialists collaborate to review individual patient cases, discuss treatment options, and formulate comprehensive care plans.

- **Decision-Making:** The tumor board enables informed decision-making by considering the unique characteristics of each patient's tumor and tailoring treatment accordingly.

3. Diagnosis and Staging:

a. Imaging and Histopathology:

- **Radiological Imaging:** Radiologists utilize various imaging modalities, such as CT scans, MRI, and PET-CT scans, to visualize the tumor's size, location, and extent.
- **Histopathological Assessment:** Pathologists analyze tissue samples obtained through biopsy or surgical resection to determine the histological subtype and molecular characteristics of the tumor.

b. Staging: Accurate staging is essential for treatment planning and prognostication. Thymic tumors are often staged using the Masaoka-Koga system for thymomas and the TNM system for thymic carcinomas.

c. The Role of Radiology and Pathology Specialists: Radiologists and pathologists play pivotal roles in providing precise imaging interpretations and histological assessments that guide treatment decisions. Their contributions are integral in achieving accurate staging and diagnosing specific subtypes of thymic tumors.

4. Treatment Planning:

a. Surgical Considerations:

- **Surgical Evaluation:** Thoracic surgeons assess the

- **Thymectomy:** The extent of thymectomy, whether it be complete or partial, is determined based on the tumor type and stage.
- **Resection Techniques:** In cases of invasive thymic carcinomas, en bloc resection may be necessary to ensure complete tumor removal.

b. Systemic Therapies:

- **Chemotherapy:** Medical oncologists administer chemotherapy, either as neoadjuvant therapy to shrink tumors before surgery or as adjuvant therapy to reduce the risk of recurrence.
- **Targeted Therapy:** For select cases with specific molecular alterations, targeted agents are considered to inhibit specific signaling pathways.
- **Immunotherapy:** Immunotherapy with immune checkpoint inhibitors is increasingly employed, particularly in advanced thymic carcinomas with high PD-L1 expression.

c. Radiation Therapy:

- **Radiation Oncologists:** These specialists plan and administer radiation therapy, which may be used preoperatively to shrink tumors, postoperatively to prevent recurrence, or as a primary treatment for inoperable cases.

5. Management of Myasthenia Gravis:

a. **Neurological Evaluation:** Neurologists evaluate and manage MG in patients with thymic tumors. MG management may include medications, such as acetylcholinesterase inhibitors or immunosuppressants.

b. Surgical Considerations: In patients with MG, thoracic surgeons may perform a thymectomy as part of MG management, even in the absence of thymic tumor symptoms.

c. Immunotherapy Impact: Immunotherapy, particularly immune checkpoint inhibitors, has shown promise in improving MG symptoms, but careful monitoring is necessary to avoid exacerbations.

6. Endocrine and Metabolic Management:

a. Endocrinologists: These specialists address endocrine abnormalities, such as hormonal imbalances or paraneoplastic syndromes associated with thymic tumors.

b. Nutritional Support: Nutritionists assist patients in maintaining optimal nutritional status, especially during chemotherapy or radiation therapy.

7. Supportive Care:

a. Palliative Care: Palliative care specialists focus on symptom management, pain control, and improving quality of life, particularly in advanced or metastatic cases.

b. Psychosocial Support: Social workers, psychologists, and counselors provide emotional and psychosocial support to patients and their families, helping them navigate the emotional challenges of a cancer diagnosis.

8. Follow-Up and Surveillance:

a. Post-Treatment Monitoring: Multidisciplinary teams collaborate in follow-up care, conducting regular assessments, imaging studies, and laboratory tests to monitor treatment response and detect recurrence.

b. Survivorship Care: Survivorship programs offer long-term care plans to address the physical and emotional needs of patients who have completed treatment.

9. Challenges and Future Directions:

a. Challenges of Rarity: The rarity of thymic tumors presents challenges in terms of limited data, expertise, and access to clinical trials.

b. Biomarker Discovery: Research is ongoing to identify reliable biomarkers that can predict treatment responses and guide therapy selection.

c. Personalized Approaches: Advancements in molecular profiling may lead to personalized treatment approaches tailored to the unique genetic characteristics of each patient's tumor.

d. Clinical Trials: Expanding participation in clinical trials for thymic tumors is essential for advancing treatment options and generating valuable data to guide future management strategies.

10. Conclusion:

A multidisciplinary approach to patient care in thymic tumors is vital for providing comprehensive and patient-centered management. The collaboration of specialists from various medical disciplines ensures that patients receive tailored treatment plans, including surgery, systemic therapies, and supportive care, addressing the unique challenges presented by thymic tumors. As research advances and the understanding of thymic tumors deepens, multidisciplinary teams play an increasingly crucial role in improving outcomes and enhancing the quality of life for patients facing these rare and complex malignancies.

5.6 Novel Therapeutic Avenues and Clinical Trials in Thymic Tumors

Advancements in the understanding of thymic tumors, driven by research and innovation, have paved the way for novel therapeutic avenues and clinical trials that hold promise for improving outcomes in patients with thymomas and thymic carcinomas. This section explores the exciting developments in the field, including emerging treatments, targeted therapies, and ongoing clinical trials, highlighting the potential to transform the landscape of thymic tumor management.

1. Novel Therapeutic Avenues:

a. The Need for Innovation: Despite progress in thymic tumor management, challenges persist, particularly in advanced or recurrent cases where conventional treatments may have limited efficacy.

b. Targeted and Personalized Approaches: Novel therapeutic avenues emphasize the importance of personalized treatment strategies based on the specific genetic and molecular characteristics of thymic tumors.

2. Targeted Therapies:

a. Molecular Profiling: The identification of genetic alterations and molecular pathways involved in thymic tumors has led to the exploration of targeted therapies tailored to individual tumor profiles.

b. Potential Targets:

- **EGFR Pathway:** Epidermal growth factor receptor (EGFR) inhibitors, such as erlotinib and gefitinib, have shown promise in tumors with EGFR mutations.

- **mTOR Pathway:** Mammalian target of rapamycin (mTOR) inhibitors, like everolimus, have been studied in thymic carcinomas.
- **PARP Inhibitors:** Poly(ADP-ribose) polymerase (PARP) inhibitors are being explored in thymic tumors with DNA repair deficiencies.

c. **Clinical Trials:** Various clinical trials are investigating the efficacy of targeted therapies either as monotherapy or in combination with other treatment modalities.

3. **Immunotherapy Advances:**

a. **Immune Checkpoint Inhibitors:** Immune checkpoint inhibitors, particularly PD-1/PD-L1 inhibitors, have shown significant promise in the treatment of thymic carcinomas with high PD-L1 expression.

b. **Combination Strategies:** Ongoing research explores combinations of immune checkpoint inhibitors with other treatment modalities, such as chemotherapy or targeted therapy, to enhance treatment responses and overcome resistance mechanisms.

c. **Predictive Biomarkers:** Identifying reliable biomarkers to predict patient responses to immunotherapy is a crucial focus of research. Biomarkers may include PD-L1 expression and other immunological factors.

4. **Emerging Therapeutic Approaches:**

a. **Antibody-Drug Conjugates (ADCs):** ADCs, which combine monoclonal antibodies with cytotoxic drugs, are being investigated as targeted therapies for thymic tumors. These agents can deliver cytotoxic payloads directly to tumor cells while sparing healthy tissue.

b. **DNA Repair Pathways:** Understanding DNA repair pathways in thymic tumors has led to the exploration of therapies that exploit vulnerabilities in these pathways. Inhibitors of DNA repair proteins are being studied for their potential to sensitize tumors to treatment.

c. Epigenetic Modifiers: Epigenetic modifications play a role in cancer development. Research into epigenetic modifiers aims to reverse these changes and restore normal gene expression in thymic tumors.

d. Tumor Microenvironment: Strategies to modulate the tumor microenvironment, such as targeting angiogenesis or immunosuppressive factors, are under investigation to enhance the efficacy of existing treatments.

5. Clinical Trials in Thymic Tumors:

a. Phase I Trials: Phase I trials assess the safety and dosage of novel therapies in a small group of patients. These trials often pave the way for further investigations.

b. Phase II Trials: Phase II trials evaluate the effectiveness and side effects of new treatments in a larger patient cohort. Promising therapies from phase I trials may advance to phase II.

c. Phase III Trials: Phase III trials compare the efficacy and safety of novel treatments with current standard treatments in a larger population. Successful phase III trials can lead to regulatory approval.

d. Ongoing Trials:

- **Targeted Therapies:** Numerous trials are investigating targeted therapies, including EGFR inhibitors, mTOR inhibitors, and PARP inhibitors.
- **Immunotherapy:** Clinical trials continue to explore immune checkpoint inhibitors and their combinations

in thymic carcinomas.

- **Novel Agents:** Ongoing trials are testing novel agents, such as antibody-drug conjugates and epigenetic modifiers.
- **Combination Therapies:** Combinations of targeted therapies, immunotherapy, and chemotherapy are being evaluated for their potential synergistic effects.

e. **Collaborative Efforts:** Multinational collaborations and academic research institutions play a vital role in conducting clinical trials in thymic tumors. These collaborative efforts facilitate patient access to cutting-edge therapies.

6. Challenges and Considerations:

a. **Rarity and Patient Enrollment:** The rarity of thymic tumors can pose challenges in patient enrollment for clinical trials. Multinational collaboration and awareness efforts are essential to ensure adequate recruitment.

b. **Biomarker Validation:** The discovery and validation of predictive biomarkers are crucial to identify patients who will benefit most from novel therapies and to spare others from potential side effects.

c. **Managing Side Effects:** Novel therapies may introduce unique side effects that require specialized management. Close monitoring and early intervention are essential for patient safety.

d. **Regulatory Approval:** The successful completion of clinical trials is a critical step in obtaining regulatory approval for novel therapies, allowing broader patient access.

7. Conclusion:

The pursuit of novel therapeutic avenues and clinical trials in thymic tumors reflects a commitment to improving the outcomes and quality of life for patients facing these rare malignancies. Targeted therapies, immunotherapy advances, and emerging therapeutic approaches offer new hope for those with thymic tumors, particularly in cases where conventional treatments have limitations. The challenges of rarity, biomarker validation, and side effect management are met with determination by researchers and healthcare professionals working collaboratively to bring innovative treatments to patients. Ongoing clinical trials, multinational collaborations, and advancements in personalized medicine are transforming the landscape of thymic tumor management, ultimately aiming to provide more effective and tailored treatments for individuals with these challenging malignancies.

CHAPTER 6: PROGNOSIS AND SURVIVAL

6.1 Predictive Factors for Outcome in Thymic Tumors

The prognosis and treatment outcomes in thymic tumors, encompassing thymomas and thymic carcinomas, can vary widely among patients. To better understand and predict the potential course of the disease, healthcare providers and researchers have identified several predictive factors that influence treatment response, disease progression, and overall survival. This section explores the critical predictive factors for outcome in thymic tumors, emphasizing the importance of personalized medicine in optimizing patient care.

1. Tumor Stage and Extent of Disease:

a. **Staging Systems:**

- **Masaoka-Koga System:** Commonly used for thymomas, this staging system considers factors such as tumor size, invasiveness, and involvement of surrounding structures.
- **TNM System:** Primarily used for thymic carcinomas, this system assesses tumor size, lymph node involvement, and metastasis.

b. **Prognostic Impact:** The stage of the tumor at diagnosis is a significant predictor of outcome. Generally, early-stage tumors (Stage I and II) have better prognoses than advanced-stage tumors (Stage III and IV).

c. Surgical Resectability: Complete surgical resection, when feasible, is associated with improved outcomes. Tumors that can be entirely removed have a higher likelihood of achieving long-term remission.

2. Histological Subtype:

a. Thymomas: Thymomas encompass a spectrum of histological subtypes, including types A, AB, B1, B2, and B3. These subtypes vary in terms of aggressiveness and likelihood of recurrence.

b. Thymic Carcinomas: Thymic carcinomas are generally considered more aggressive than thymomas, with a higher potential for metastasis and recurrence.

c. Prognostic Variability: The histological subtype is a significant prognostic factor, with type B3 thymomas and thymic carcinomas typically associated with poorer outcomes compared to other thymoma subtypes.

3. Molecular and Genetic Alterations:

a. Molecular Profiling: Advances in molecular profiling have revealed specific genetic alterations in thymic tumors that can influence treatment response and prognosis.

b. Examples of Molecular Alterations:

- **EGFR Mutations:** Thymic carcinomas with EGFR mutations may respond favorably to EGFR inhibitors.
- **DNA Repair Deficiencies:** Tumors with DNA repair deficiencies may exhibit sensitivity to therapies targeting these pathways.

- **PD-L1 Expression:** High PD-L1 expression is associated with better responses to immune checkpoint inhibitors.

c. **Personalized Treatment:** Identifying molecular alterations in individual tumors allows for personalized treatment strategies, targeting specific genetic vulnerabilities.

4. Myasthenia Gravis (MG) and Autoimmune Disorders:

a. **Association with MG:** Thymic tumors are often associated with MG, an autoimmune neuromuscular disorder. The presence of MG can complicate treatment and influence outcomes.

b. **MG Management:** Effective management of MG, whether through medical therapy or thymectomy, can improve patient outcomes and quality of life.

c. **Impact on Prognosis:** The presence of MG can affect the course of thymic tumor treatment and may influence the choice of therapeutic modalities.

5. Age and Performance Status:

a. **Age:** Patient age can impact treatment decisions and tolerance of therapies. Older patients may have comorbidities that affect treatment choices.

b. **Performance Status:** The Eastern Cooperative Oncology Group (ECOG) performance status is often used to assess a patient's overall health and functional status. A lower performance status may indicate a reduced ability to tolerate aggressive treatments.

c. **Prognostic Significance:** Younger age and a better performance status are generally associated with improved treatment outcomes.

6. Immune Checkpoint Expression:

a. PD-L1 Expression: High expression of programmed death-ligand 1 (PD-L1) on tumor cells may predict better responses to immune checkpoint inhibitors, particularly in thymic carcinomas.

b. Predictive Biomarker: PD-L1 expression serves as a potential predictive biomarker for immunotherapy response in thymic tumors.

7. Surgical Margins and Residual Disease:

a. Surgical Resection: The extent of surgical resection and the achievement of clear surgical margins influence prognosis. Complete resection with negative margins is associated with better outcomes.

b. Residual Disease: Residual tumor after surgery, known as microscopic or macroscopic residual disease, is a negative prognostic factor and may necessitate adjuvant therapies.

8. Tumor Growth Rate and Response to Neoadjuvant Therapy:

a. Tumor Growth Rate: Rapidly growing tumors may have a worse prognosis compared to slow-growing tumors.

b. Neoadjuvant Therapy Response: The response of thymic tumors to neoadjuvant therapy, such as chemotherapy or targeted agents, can provide valuable prognostic information.

9. Metastasis and Lymph Node Involvement:

a. Distant Metastasis: The presence of distant metastases at diagnosis, such as lung or bone involvement, typically indicates a more advanced stage and poorer prognosis.

b. Lymph Node Involvement: Lymph node metastasis, especially in thymic carcinomas, is associated with a higher likelihood of disease recurrence and a more aggressive disease course.

10. Adjuvant and Salvage Therapies:

a. Adjuvant Therapies: The use of adjuvant therapies, such as radiation or chemotherapy after surgical resection, can impact long-term outcomes.

b. Salvage Therapies: Salvage therapies for recurrent or refractory disease may offer the potential for disease control and prolonged survival.

11. Compliance and Tolerance to Treatment:

a. Treatment Compliance: Patient adherence to treatment regimens is crucial for achieving optimal outcomes. Missed treatments or noncompliance can impact treatment efficacy.

b. Treatment Tolerance: The ability to tolerate treatment, including the management of side effects, is essential for maintaining quality of life during therapy.

12. Multidisciplinary Care and Expertise:

a. Role of Multidisciplinary Teams: The involvement of multidisciplinary teams with expertise in thymic tumors can lead to more informed treatment decisions and improved patient outcomes.

b. Centers of Excellence: Treatment at specialized centers with experience in managing thymic tumors can lead to better outcomes due to access to the latest therapies and clinical trials.

13. Future Directions:

a. **Biomarker Discovery:** Ongoing research aims to identify additional predictive biomarkers, including genetic, molecular, and immunological factors, to refine treatment strategies further.

b. **Personalized Medicine:** The future of thymic tumor management lies in personalized medicine, where treatments are tailored to the specific characteristics of each patient's tumor.

c. **Clinical Trials:** Participation in clinical trials is critical for advancing our understanding of thymic tumors and discovering new predictive factors and treatments.

14. Conclusion:

Predictive factors for outcome in thymic tumors play a pivotal role in guiding treatment decisions, individualizing therapy, and providing prognostic information to patients and their healthcare teams. The integration of these predictive factors, such as tumor stage, histological subtype, molecular profile, and patient-related factors, allows for a comprehensive assessment of the disease and helps optimize treatment approaches. As ongoing research continues to uncover new predictive factors and refine existing ones, the goal remains to improve the prognosis and quality of life for individuals facing the challenges of thymic tumors through personalized and evidence-based care.

6.2 Survival Rates and Long-Term Follow-Up in Thymic Tumors

Understanding the survival rates and implementing long-term follow-up strategies are crucial components of managing thymic tumors, encompassing thymomas and thymic carcinomas. These rare malignancies, originating in the thymus gland, exhibit diverse clinical behaviors and require tailored approaches to treatment and surveillance. This section explores the survival rates associated with thymic tumors, the factors influencing them, and the importance of long-term follow-up care for patients.

1. Overview of Thymic Tumors:

a. Rarity: Thymic tumors are rare, accounting for only a small percentage of mediastinal neoplasms. Their rarity can pose challenges in data collection and research.

b. Heterogeneity: Thymic tumors exhibit a wide range of histological subtypes, each with distinct clinical characteristics and outcomes.

2. Survival Rates in Thymic Tumors:

a. Five-Year Survival Rates: Survival rates in thymic tumors vary depending on factors such as histological subtype, stage at diagnosis, and treatment received. However, five-year survival rates provide a general overview of outcomes.

b. Thymomas: Five-year survival rates for thymomas range from approximately 50% to 95%, with early-stage, resectable thymomas having higher survival rates.

c. Thymic Carcinomas: Thymic carcinomas generally have lower five-year survival rates, ranging from approximately 20% to 70%, largely due to their aggressive nature and frequent presentation at advanced stages.

d. Recurrent and Metastatic Disease: Patients with recurrent or metastatic thymic tumors often have poorer survival rates than those with localized disease.

3. Factors Influencing Survival:

a. Stage at Diagnosis: The stage of the tumor at diagnosis is a critical determinant of survival. Early-stage tumors typically have better outcomes than advanced-stage tumors.

b. Histological Subtype: The histological subtype of the tumor significantly influences prognosis. Some thymoma subtypes have more favorable outcomes than others, while thymic carcinomas are generally associated with lower survival rates.

c. Resectability: Complete surgical resection with negative margins is associated with improved survival, particularly in thymomas.

d. Adjuvant Therapies: The use of adjuvant therapies, such as radiation therapy or chemotherapy after surgery, can impact long-term outcomes.

e. Response to Treatment: The response of thymic tumors to treatment, including chemotherapy, targeted therapy, and immunotherapy, can affect survival rates.

f. Age and Comorbidities: Patient age and the presence of comorbidities can influence treatment options, tolerance, and ultimately, survival.

4. Importance of Long-Term Follow-Up:

a. Surveillance and Monitoring: Long-term follow-up care is essential to monitor for disease recurrence, assess treatment-related side effects, and address the ongoing health needs of thymic tumor survivors.

b. Detection of Recurrence: Thymic tumors, particularly thymomas, can exhibit late recurrences, underscoring the importance of prolonged surveillance.

c. Surveillance Imaging: Regular imaging studies, such as chest CT scans and PET-CT scans, are conducted to detect any signs of recurrence or metastasis.

d. **Functional Assessments:** Assessments of lung function and cardiac function may be necessary, especially in patients who have undergone extensive surgical resections.

e. **Evaluation of Myasthenia Gravis:** Patients with MG require ongoing evaluation and management to address MG-related symptoms, which may change over time.

5. **Challenges in Long-Term Follow-Up:**

a. **Rarity of Thymic Tumors:** The rarity of thymic tumors can make it challenging for healthcare providers to develop standardized follow-up protocols and guidelines.

b. **Late Recurrences:** Thymomas are known for late recurrences, sometimes occurring decades after initial treatment, necessitating prolonged surveillance.

c. **Multidisciplinary Approach:** A multidisciplinary approach, involving oncologists, surgeons, radiologists, and other specialists, is essential for comprehensive long-term follow-up care.

6. **Follow-Up Strategies and Guidelines:**

a. **Surveillance Schedules:** Follow-up schedules may vary based on individual patient characteristics, but they often involve regular visits and imaging at specified intervals.

b. **Imaging Modalities:** Chest CT scans and PET-CT scans are commonly used imaging modalities for surveillance, with the frequency of scans depending on the patient's risk profile.

c. **Functional Assessments:** Pulmonary function tests (PFTs) and cardiac assessments may be performed as needed, especially in patients with a history of extensive surgery.

d. **MG Evaluation:** Patients with MG require ongoing

evaluations to monitor their neurological symptoms and MG status.

7. Survivorship Care:

a. Survivorship Programs: Survivorship programs focus on addressing the long-term physical and emotional needs of thymic tumor survivors.

b. Quality of Life: Enhancing the quality of life for survivors includes managing treatment-related side effects, providing psychosocial support, and promoting healthy lifestyle behaviors.

c. Management of Late Effects: Survivorship care teams are equipped to manage late effects of treatment, including cardiac issues, secondary malignancies, and other complications.

8. Research and Future Directions:

a. Improved Risk Stratification: Ongoing research aims to refine risk stratification and develop more precise predictive models for thymic tumor outcomes.

b. Novel Therapies: Advancements in targeted therapies and immunotherapies offer new treatment options that may impact long-term survival rates.

c. Late Recurrence Studies: Research on the factors contributing to late recurrences in thymomas may lead to better strategies for detection and prevention.

d. Survivorship Research: Investigating survivorship issues and quality of life concerns is an integral part of thymic tumor research.

9. Conclusion:

Survival rates and long-term follow-up care are integral components of managing thymic tumors. While outcomes can vary widely based on factors such as stage, histological subtype, and treatment response, ongoing research and multidisciplinary care have the potential to improve survival rates and enhance the quality of life for thymic tumor survivors. The rarity of these malignancies underscores the importance of specialized care and long-term surveillance to detect recurrence and address the unique challenges associated with thymic tumors. Ultimately, the goal is to provide personalized, evidence-based care that optimizes long-term outcomes and survivorship for individuals facing thymic tumors.

6.3 Recurrence Patterns and Management in Thymic Tumors

Recurrence is a significant concern in the management of thymic tumors, encompassing thymomas and thymic carcinomas. While some patients achieve remission after initial treatment, others may experience disease recurrence, which can be challenging to manage. This section explores the recurrence patterns, risk factors, and strategies for the management of recurrent thymic tumors.

1. Recurrence Patterns in Thymic Tumors:

a. Timing of Recurrence: Recurrence in thymic tumors can occur at various time points:

- **Early Recurrence:** Recurrence within the first few years after initial treatment.
- **Late Recurrence:** Recurrence that manifests years or even decades after the initial treatment, especially in thymomas.

b. Local vs. Distant Recurrence: Recurrence may be local (within the mediastinum) or distant, often in the lungs, bones, or other organs.

c. Histological Subtype: The histological subtype of the thymic tumor can influence recurrence patterns. For instance, type B3 thymomas and thymic carcinomas tend to have a higher risk of recurrence.

d. Residual Disease: Incomplete surgical resection or microscopic residual disease after surgery can increase the risk of recurrence.

e. Myasthenia Gravis (MG): MG status may also impact recurrence patterns, as some MG-associated thymomas exhibit more aggressive behavior.

2. Risk Factors for Recurrence:

a. Tumor Stage: Advanced-stage tumors (Stage III and IV) are more likely to recur than early-stage tumors (Stage I and II).

b. Surgical Margins: Incomplete surgical resection or positive surgical margins increase the risk of local recurrence.

c. Lymph Node Involvement: Lymph node metastasis is associated with a higher likelihood of recurrence, particularly in thymic carcinomas.

d. Histological Subtype: Some histological subtypes, such as type B3 thymomas and thymic carcinomas, have a greater propensity for recurrence.

e. Adjuvant Therapies: The absence of adjuvant therapies, such as radiation therapy or chemotherapy, in high-risk cases may contribute to recurrence.

f. Response to Initial Treatment: Poor response to initial treatment, including inadequate response to chemotherapy or targeted therapy, may lead to disease persistence and recurrence.

g. Myasthenia Gravis (MG): MG status can influence recurrence patterns, as thymomas associated with MG may exhibit different behavior.

3. Strategies for Recurrence Management:

a. Local Recurrence:

i. Surgical Resection: In cases of local recurrence within the mediastinum, surgical resection may be considered if feasible and if the patient's overall health allows.

ii. Radiation Therapy: Radiation therapy may be used to manage localized recurrence, especially when surgery is not an option or in cases of positive surgical margins.

iii. Salvage Chemotherapy: Salvage chemotherapy regimens can be employed to target recurrent disease, often in combination with other modalities.

b. Distant Metastases:

i. Systemic Therapies: For distant metastases, systemic therapies such as chemotherapy, targeted therapy, or immunotherapy may be employed to control the spread of the disease.

ii. Molecular Profiling: Molecular profiling of the recurrent tumor can help identify targeted therapies that may be effective in controlling the disease.

c. Multidisciplinary Approach:

i. Multidisciplinary Tumor Boards: A multidisciplinary approach, involving tumor boards with specialists in oncology, surgery, radiation therapy, and pathology, is crucial for designing individualized management plans.

ii. Clinical Trials: Participation in clinical trials exploring novel therapies for recurrent thymic tumors is an option to consider.

d. Surveillance and Follow-Up:

i. Regular Imaging: Close surveillance with regular imaging studies is essential to monitor for recurrent disease or progression.

ii. Functional Assessments: Pulmonary and cardiac assessments may be necessary to evaluate the impact of recurrent disease on organ function.

e. Supportive Care:

i. Symptom Management: Addressing symptoms related to disease recurrence, such as pain or shortness of breath, is an essential aspect of care.

ii. Psychological Support: Patients facing recurrence often require psychological support to cope with the emotional impact of the disease.

f. Quality of Life Considerations:

i. Survivorship Programs: Engaging patients in survivorship programs can help manage the long-term physical and emotional aspects of living with recurrent thymic tumors.

ii. Palliative Care: In cases where the disease is advanced or untreatable, palliative care focuses on enhancing the patient's quality of life and managing symptoms.

4. Challenges in Recurrence Management:

a. Limited Treatment Options: Recurrent thymic tumors can be challenging to treat, especially when standard treatment options have been exhausted.

b. Rarity of Thymic Tumors: The rarity of thymic tumors means that evidence-based guidelines for managing recurrence are limited, necessitating a personalized approach.

c. Late Recurrences: Late recurrences, particularly in thymomas, can be unexpected and difficult to detect, emphasizing the need for prolonged surveillance.

d. Multidisciplinary Care: Coordinating care across multiple specialties in recurrent cases can be complex but is essential for comprehensive management.

5. Survivorship and Long-Term Follow-Up:

a. Long-Term Surveillance: Patients with recurrent thymic tumors often require long-term surveillance to monitor disease status and evaluate treatment responses.

b. Survivorship Care Plans: Survivorship care plans outline the necessary follow-up care, including imaging schedules, functional assessments, and symptom management.

c. Quality of Life: The focus of long-term care is not only on disease management but also on improving the patient's quality of life and addressing any late effects of treatment.

6. Research and Future Directions:

a. Targeted Therapies: Ongoing research aims to identify targeted therapies that can effectively control recurrent thymic tumors, particularly those with specific molecular alterations.

b. Immunotherapy: Investigational studies exploring the role of immunotherapy in managing recurrent thymic tumors are ongoing.

c. Survivorship Research: Research on survivorship issues, including late effects and psychological well-being, is integral to improving the long-term care of patients with recurrent thymic tumors.

7. Conclusion:

Managing recurrence in thymic tumors is a complex and individualized process that requires a multidisciplinary approach, close surveillance, and consideration of patient-specific factors. While recurrent thymic tumors can present challenges, ongoing research and advancements in targeted therapy and immunotherapy offer hope for improved outcomes and enhanced quality of life for patients facing recurrence. The rarity of these malignancies underscores the importance of specialized care and comprehensive long-term follow-up to detect and manage recurrence effectively. Ultimately, the goal is to provide personalized, evidence-based care that optimizes the management of recurrent thymic tumors and enhances the well-being of affected individuals.

6.4 Quality of Life and Survivorship Issues in Thymic Tumors

Surviving thymic tumors, including thymomas and thymic carcinomas, is a significant achievement, but it often comes with physical, emotional, and social challenges. Quality of life and survivorship issues are essential aspects of the long-term care of patients who have undergone treatment for these rare malignancies. This section explores the impact of thymic tumors on quality of life, survivorship concerns, and strategies for addressing the unique needs of survivors.

1. Quality of Life in Thymic Tumor Survivors:

a. Physical Well-being: Thymic tumor survivors may experience physical challenges related to their disease or treatment. These can include:

- **Surgical Effects:** Persistent pain, scarring, and changes in lung or heart function following surgery.
- **Fatigue:** Fatigue may persist even after treatment completion.
- **Respiratory Symptoms:** Breathing difficulties or coughing may affect daily life.
- **Cardiac Issues:** Radiation therapy or surgical procedures can impact cardiac health.

b. Emotional Well-being: Survivors may experience a range of emotions, including anxiety, depression, and fear of recurrence. The emotional impact of the disease can be profound.

c. Social and Occupational Impacts: The challenges of treatment and lingering symptoms may affect social relationships and employment. Some survivors may face difficulties in returning to work or maintaining their usual activities.

d. Myasthenia Gravis (MG): MG-associated thymomas add another layer of complexity to survivors' quality of life, as the autoimmune disorder may persist or fluctuate.

2. Survivorship Concerns in Thymic Tumors:

a. Late Recurrence: Thymoma survivors face the possibility of late recurrences, sometimes decades after initial treatment, which can be emotionally distressing.

b. Long-Term Surveillance: Survivors require ongoing surveillance to monitor for disease recurrence, which may necessitate regular imaging studies and clinical assessments.

c. Late Effects of Treatment: Late effects of treatment, such as cardiac issues, secondary malignancies, or neurological symptoms, may emerge years after treatment completion.

d. Psychological Distress: The fear of recurrence and the emotional toll of a cancer diagnosis can lead to psychological distress and impact the survivor's overall well-being.

e. Changes in Body Image: Surgical scars and changes in physical appearance may affect body image and self-esteem.

f. Coping with MG: Thymoma survivors with MG need ongoing management of their autoimmune disorder, which can be unpredictable and impact daily life.

3. Strategies for Improving Quality of Life and Addressing Survivorship Issues:

a. Survivorship Care Plans:

i. Survivorship Care Teams: Specialized survivorship care teams comprised of oncologists, nurses, social workers, and psychologists play a crucial role in addressing survivorship concerns.

ii. Survivorship Care Plans: Individualized survivorship care plans outline follow-up schedules, surveillance protocols, and strategies for managing late effects and psychological distress.

b. Physical Rehabilitation:

i. Pulmonary Rehabilitation: For survivors with breathing difficulties, pulmonary rehabilitation programs can help improve lung function and alleviate symptoms.

ii. Cardiac Rehabilitation: Survivors with cardiac issues may benefit from cardiac rehabilitation programs to enhance heart health.

c. Supportive Care:

i. Symptom Management: Effective symptom management,

including pain control and relief from treatment-related side effects, is essential for improving quality of life.

ii. Psychological Support: Survivors may benefit from psychological support, including counseling or support groups, to address emotional distress and fears related to recurrence.

d. Survivorship Research:

i. Late Effects Studies: Research on late effects of thymic tumor treatment is essential for understanding and mitigating potential long-term complications.

ii. Quality of Life Research: Investigating the factors that influence quality of life in thymic tumor survivors can guide interventions to enhance well-being.

e. Multidisciplinary Care:

i. Coordination of Care: A multidisciplinary approach ensures that survivors receive comprehensive care addressing their physical, emotional, and social needs.

ii. Specialty Clinics: Some healthcare centers offer specialty survivorship clinics where survivors can access a range of services and support.

f. Rehabilitation and Lifestyle Interventions:

i. Physical Activity: Encouraging survivors to engage in regular physical activity can improve physical and emotional well-being.

ii. Diet and Nutrition: Nutritional counseling can help survivors maintain a healthy diet and manage any treatment-related dietary restrictions.

g. Managing Late Effects:

i. Cardiac Monitoring: Survivors at risk of cardiac issues require ongoing monitoring and management, which may include medications or lifestyle modifications.

ii. Secondary Malignancy Screening: Survivors may need regular screenings for secondary malignancies, especially if they received radiation therapy.

4. Coping with Myasthenia Gravis:

a. MG Management: For thymoma survivors with MG, ongoing management of the autoimmune disorder is essential. This may involve medications, immunosuppressive therapies, or plasmapheresis.

b. Neurological Assessments: Regular assessments by neurologists are necessary to monitor MG-related neurological symptoms and adjust treatment as needed.

5. Survivorship Programs and Resources:

a. Survivorship Programs: Many cancer centers offer survivorship programs that provide a range of services, including counseling, support groups, and educational resources.

b. Online Communities: Online communities and support groups can connect survivors with others facing similar challenges, offering a sense of camaraderie and shared experiences.

c. Educational Materials: Educational materials and resources on thymic tumors and survivorship issues empower survivors with knowledge about their condition and available support.

6. Future Directions:

a. Survivorship Research: Research in thymic tumor

survivorship is ongoing, with a focus on improving our understanding of long-term outcomes and enhancing survivorship care.

b. Late Effects Management: Continued research into the management of late effects and strategies to mitigate their impact is crucial.

c. Psychosocial Support: Enhanced psychosocial support services and interventions will help survivors cope with the emotional challenges of living with thymic tumors.

7. Conclusion:

Quality of life and survivorship concerns in thymic tumor survivors are multifaceted and require a holistic approach to care. Survivorship care plans, multidisciplinary teams, and specialized support services are essential components of addressing the unique needs of survivors. As research advances and survivorship care evolves, the goal is to optimize the quality of life for individuals who have triumphed over thymic tumors, providing them with the resources and support needed to lead fulfilling lives beyond their cancer journey.

6.5 Supportive Care and Palliative Strategies in Thymic Tumors

Supportive care and palliative strategies play an integral role in the comprehensive management of thymic tumors, encompassing thymomas and thymic carcinomas. While medical interventions focus on treating the disease, supportive care and palliative measures aim to enhance the overall well-being of patients, alleviate symptoms, and improve their quality of life. This section explores the importance of supportive care and palliative strategies in the context of thymic tumors.

1. Understanding Supportive Care and Palliative Care:

a. Supportive Care: Supportive care refers to a broad range of medical, emotional, and psychological interventions designed to improve the quality of life for patients facing a serious illness, such as thymic tumors. It can be integrated into the patient's treatment plan from the time of diagnosis and continues throughout the cancer journey.

b. Palliative Care: Palliative care is a specialized form of supportive care that focuses on providing relief from the symptoms, pain, and emotional distress associated with serious illnesses. It can be initiated at any stage of the disease, including alongside curative treatments.

2. The Role of Supportive Care in Thymic Tumors:

a. Symptom Management: Supportive care addresses the numerous symptoms that patients with thymic tumors may experience, such as pain, shortness of breath, fatigue, and psychological distress.

b. Side Effect Management: Patients undergoing treatments like surgery, radiation, or chemotherapy may experience side effects, such as nausea, vomiting, and immunosuppression. Supportive care helps manage these side effects.

c. Psychological Support: The emotional toll of a thymic tumor diagnosis can be significant. Supportive care includes counseling, therapy, and psychosocial support to help patients and their families cope with the psychological impact of the disease.

d. Nutritional Support: For patients who experience appetite changes or difficulty eating, nutritional support ensures that they receive adequate nourishment to maintain their strength and stamina.

e. Physical Rehabilitation: Patients who have undergone surgery or experienced physical deconditioning may benefit from physical therapy and rehabilitation to regain their functional capacity.

f. Complementary Therapies: Supportive care often incorporates complementary therapies such as acupuncture, massage, and relaxation techniques to manage symptoms and improve well-being.

3. Palliative Care in Thymic Tumors:

a. Pain Management: Palliative care plays a crucial role in addressing pain associated with thymic tumors, offering various strategies for pain relief, including medications, nerve blocks, and other interventions.

b. End-of-Life Care: In advanced stages of thymic tumors, palliative care focuses on providing comfort and dignity to patients nearing the end of life. This may involve hospice care and addressing end-of-life decisions.

c. Symptom Relief: Palliative care professionals are skilled in symptom management, offering solutions for symptom relief, such as dyspnea (shortness of breath) management and treatment for cancer-related fatigue.

d. Emotional and Spiritual Support: Palliative care addresses the emotional and spiritual needs of patients and their families, providing guidance on difficult conversations and end-of-life planning.

e. Holistic Approach: Palliative care adopts a holistic approach that considers the physical, emotional, psychological, and spiritual aspects of a patient's well-being.

4. The Multidisciplinary Approach:

a. Collaborative Care Teams: The integration of supportive care and palliative care into the treatment of thymic tumors requires a collaborative approach involving oncologists, palliative care specialists, nurses, social workers, psychologists, and other healthcare professionals.

b. Communication: Effective communication between the patient, family, and the healthcare team is essential to tailor supportive and palliative care to the patient's individual needs and preferences.

5. Decision-Making and Advance Care Planning:

a. Shared Decision-Making: Shared decision-making involves patients, their families, and healthcare providers collaborating to make informed choices about treatment options, goals of care, and advance care planning.

b. Advance Directives: Patients with thymic tumors are encouraged to create advance directives, which specify their preferences for medical care, including decisions regarding life-sustaining treatments and end-of-life care.

6. Survivorship and Supportive Care:

a. Survivorship Programs: Survivorship programs provide long-term support to thymic tumor survivors, addressing not only the physical but also the psychological and emotional aspects of survivorship.

b. Quality of Life: Supportive care continues to play a crucial role in the post-treatment phase, focusing on improving the survivor's quality of life and addressing late effects.

7. Challenges in Supportive and Palliative Care:

a. Recognizing the Need: Recognizing the need for supportive and palliative care in thymic tumors can sometimes be challenging, as patients and families may focus primarily on curative treatments.

b. Access to Care: Access to supportive and palliative care services may vary depending on the healthcare setting, geographic location, and availability of specialized professionals.

c. Cultural and Psychological Barriers: Cultural beliefs, stigmas, and psychological barriers may affect a patient's willingness to accept and engage with supportive and palliative care.

d. Care Coordination: Effective coordination between the oncology team and supportive and palliative care specialists is essential to ensure that care plans align with the patient's goals and preferences.

8. Future Directions in Supportive and Palliative Care:

a. Research: Ongoing research aims to better understand the impact of supportive and palliative care interventions on the well-being and outcomes of thymic tumor patients.

b. Integration of Care: The integration of supportive and palliative care into routine oncology practice is a focus of future initiatives, aiming to improve the quality of care and patient experience.

c. Education and Training: Training healthcare providers in supportive and palliative care is essential to ensure that all patients with thymic tumors have access to these vital services.

d. Patient-Centered Approaches: Future developments should prioritize patient-centered approaches that empower patients to make informed decisions about their care and quality of life.

9. Conclusion:

Supportive care and palliative strategies are integral components of the holistic care provided to thymic tumor patients. Recognizing the importance of addressing the physical, emotional, and psychological needs of patients and their families can significantly enhance the overall well-being and quality of life of individuals facing these rare malignancies. As the field of supportive and palliative care continues to evolve, the goal is to ensure that all thymic tumor patients receive the comprehensive care they need to navigate their cancer journey with dignity, comfort, and improved quality of life.

6.6 Survivorship Care Plans in Thymic Tumors

Survivorship care plans (SCPs) are essential tools in the comprehensive management of thymic tumors, encompassing thymomas and thymic carcinomas. These personalized documents outline the individualized follow-up care, surveillance protocols, and strategies to address the unique needs and concerns of thymic tumor survivors. In this section, we explore the importance of survivorship care plans and their role in optimizing the long-term well-being of individuals who have triumphed over thymic tumors.

1. Survivorship Care Plans:

a. **Definition:** Survivorship care plans (SCPs) are comprehensive, individualized documents that summarize a patient's cancer history, treatment received, potential late effects, and provide recommendations for ongoing follow-up care and support.

b. **Purpose:** SCPs serve several critical purposes, including:

- **Facilitating Communication:** SCPs promote communication between patients, their primary care

providers, and oncology teams.
- **Guiding Follow-Up Care:** They provide clear guidelines for follow-up care, surveillance, and screening.
- **Addressing Late Effects:** SCPs help anticipate and address potential late effects of cancer treatment.
- **Empowering Patients:** They empower survivors to take an active role in their long-term care and advocate for their needs.

2. Creating Survivorship Care Plans for Thymic Tumors:

a. Individualized Approach: SCPs for thymic tumors should be highly individualized, considering factors such as tumor stage, treatment modalities, histological subtype, and the presence of Myasthenia Gravis (MG).

b. Involvement of Multidisciplinary Teams: The development of SCPs often involves a multidisciplinary team, including oncologists, surgeons, radiation oncologists, nurses, social workers, and psychologists.

c. Survivorship Care Coordinator: Some healthcare centers employ survivorship care coordinators who guide patients through the creation of their SCPs, ensuring that all aspects of care are addressed.

3. Components of a Thymic Tumor Survivorship Care Plan:

a. Diagnosis and Treatment Summary:

i. Diagnosis: Include details of the thymic tumor diagnosis, including histological subtype and stage.

ii. Treatment History: Summarize the treatment received, such as surgery, radiation therapy, chemotherapy, targeted therapy, and immunotherapy.

b. Follow-Up Schedule:

i. Surveillance: Outline the recommended schedule for surveillance, including the frequency of imaging studies (e.g., CT scans, PET-CT scans) and clinical assessments.

ii. Functional Assessments: Specify when and how pulmonary and cardiac function assessments should be conducted.

iii. MG Monitoring: If applicable, detail the schedule for MG monitoring, including neurological assessments.

c. Late Effects Management:

i. Potential Late Effects: Identify potential late effects of thymic tumor treatment, such as cardiac issues, secondary malignancies, and psychological distress.

ii. Strategies for Management: Describe strategies for monitoring and managing late effects, including medications, lifestyle modifications, and psychosocial support.

d. Psychosocial Support:

i. Emotional Well-being: Highlight the importance of addressing emotional and psychological concerns, and provide resources for counseling or support groups.

ii. Coping Strategies: Offer guidance on coping with the emotional impact of cancer survivorship and provide information on stress-reduction techniques.

e. Lifestyle Recommendations:

i. Physical Activity: Encourage survivors to engage in regular physical activity and provide guidance on safe exercise routines.

ii. Diet and Nutrition: Offer dietary recommendations, especially if there are specific dietary considerations related to treatment.

f. Sexual Health and Fertility:

i. Fertility Preservation: If applicable, discuss fertility preservation options and family planning considerations.

ii. Sexual Health: Provide information on maintaining sexual health and addressing sexual concerns.

g. Advance Care Planning:

i. Advance Directives: Encourage the completion of advance directives to ensure that a patient's preferences for medical care are known and respected.

ii. Goals of Care: Discuss the patient's goals of care, including preferences for aggressive treatment, symptom management, and end-of-life care.

h. Resources and Support:

i. Supportive Services: List resources for patients and caregivers, including organizations, support groups, and financial assistance programs.

ii. Contact Information: Provide contact information for the survivorship care coordinator or point of contact for questions and concerns.

4. Importance of Survivorship Care Plans in Thymic Tumors:

a. Long-Term Follow-Up: SCPs ensure that survivors receive appropriate long-term follow-up care, which is essential for detecting recurrence and managing late effects.

b. Continuity of Care: They facilitate seamless transitions from oncology care to primary care, ensuring that survivors' health needs are addressed comprehensively.

c. Empowerment: SCPs empower survivors to take an active role in their health and advocate for their needs, promoting a sense of control and self-efficacy.

d. Addressing Late Effects: SCPs proactively address the potential late effects of thymic tumor treatment, allowing for early detection and intervention.

e. Communication: SCPs enhance communication between patients and healthcare providers, fostering a collaborative approach to care.

f. Quality of Life: By addressing physical, emotional, and psychosocial aspects of survivorship, SCPs contribute to improving the overall quality of life for thymic tumor survivors.

5. Challenges in Implementing Survivorship Care Plans:

a. Awareness: Not all patients and healthcare providers are aware of the importance of SCPs, which can hinder their implementation.

b. Access to Survivorship Care: Access to specialized survivorship care and survivorship care coordinators may be limited in certain healthcare settings.

c. Survivorship Needs: Meeting the diverse needs of thymic tumor survivors can be challenging due to the rarity of these malignancies and the variability in treatment approaches.

d. Coordination: Effective coordination between oncology teams, primary care providers, and other specialists is essential for implementing SCPs.

6. Future Directions in Survivorship Care:

a. Personalized Medicine: Advancements in personalized

medicine may lead to more tailored survivorship care plans based on genetic and molecular characteristics.

b. Survivorship Research: Ongoing research aims to improve our understanding of survivorship issues in thymic tumors and develop evidence-based interventions.

c. Telehealth: Telehealth and digital tools may play a growing role in delivering survivorship care and providing resources to survivors.

d. Survivorship Education: Efforts to educate both patients and healthcare providers about the importance of SCPs and survivorship care are essential.

7. Conclusion:

Survivorship care plans are invaluable tools in the long-term care of individuals who have overcome thymic tumors. They offer a roadmap for follow-up care, surveillance, and addressing the unique needs of survivors, encompassing physical, emotional, and psychosocial aspects of survivorship. As the field of survivorship care continues to evolve, the goal is to ensure that all thymic tumor survivors have access to personalized, comprehensive care plans that empower them to live healthy, fulfilling

CHAPTER 7: THYMIC TUMORS IN PEDIATRICS

7.1 Pediatric Thymic Tumors: Epidemiology and Characteristics

Pediatric thymic tumors, although rare, present a unique set of challenges and considerations compared to their adult counterparts. This section delves into the epidemiology, characteristics, clinical presentation, and management of thymic tumors in the pediatric population, shedding light on this less common but significant medical condition.

Thymic tumors are exceptionally rare in children, accounting for only a small fraction of all pediatric malignancies. Unlike adult thymic tumors, which typically occur in the anterior mediastinum, pediatric thymic tumors can manifest in various locations within the mediastinum, making their diagnosis and management even more complex.

2. Epidemiology:

a. Incidence: Pediatric thymic tumors are extremely uncommon, with an estimated annual incidence of fewer than 0.5 cases per million children.

b. Age Distribution: These tumors can occur across a wide age range in the pediatric population, but they are most frequently diagnosed during adolescence.

c. Gender: Thymic tumors in children show no significant gender predilection, affecting both males and females equally.

d. Association with Myasthenia Gravis: Unlike adult thymomas, pediatric thymic tumors are rarely associated with Myasthenia Gravis (MG), an autoimmune neuromuscular disorder. MG is more commonly seen in adults with thymic tumors.

3. Classification and Histological Subtypes:

Pediatric thymic tumors encompass a spectrum of histological subtypes, similar to those seen in adults. The most common histological subtypes include:

a. Thymomas: These are the most prevalent pediatric thymic tumors. Thymomas are characterized by a varied range of cellular compositions, and they are further classified into different subtypes based on their histology (e.g., type A, AB, B1, B2, B3).

b. Thymic Carcinomas: Thymic carcinomas are a more aggressive form of thymic tumor and are less common in children than thymomas.

c. Thymic Neuroendocrine Tumors: These tumors, which may include carcinoid tumors, are exceedingly rare in the pediatric population.

d. Thymic Cysts: Benign thymic cysts can also occur in children and are typically non-cancerous.

4. Clinical Presentation:

Pediatric thymic tumors often present with a spectrum of symptoms, which may include:

a. Chest Pain: Pain or discomfort in the chest region may be a presenting symptom, although it is nonspecific.

b. Cough and Respiratory Symptoms: Children may experience cough, shortness of breath, and recurrent respiratory infections due to the mass effect of the tumor within the mediastinum.

c. Superior Vena Cava Syndrome: In rare cases, large thymic tumors can compress the superior vena cava, leading to symptoms such as facial swelling, dilated neck veins, and upper body edema.

d. Myasthenia Gravis: While uncommon, pediatric thymic tumors can be associated with MG, which can manifest as muscle weakness, drooping eyelids, and difficulty swallowing or breathing.

e. Asymptomatic: Some pediatric thymic tumors are discovered incidentally during imaging studies performed for unrelated reasons, such as chest X-rays or CT scans.

5. Diagnosis and Evaluation:

a. Imaging: Radiological imaging, such as chest X-rays, CT scans, or MRI scans, is often employed to visualize the tumor's size, location, and extent within the mediastinum.

b. Biopsy: A definitive diagnosis of pediatric thymic tumors typically requires a tissue biopsy, which can be obtained through minimally invasive procedures like needle biopsy or open surgical biopsy.

c. Histopathology: Once a biopsy is performed, histopathological examination determines the tumor's subtype and grade, guiding treatment decisions.

d. Myasthenia Gravis Evaluation: When associated with MG, pediatric patients may undergo specific tests to confirm the autoimmune disorder.

e. Staging: Staging assessments help determine the tumor's extent and guide treatment planning. Staging may include imaging studies and sometimes surgical exploration.

6. Treatment Modalities:

The management of pediatric thymic tumors requires a multidisciplinary approach, involving pediatric oncologists, surgeons, radiation oncologists, and other specialists. Treatment options may include:

a. Surgery: Surgical resection is often the primary treatment for localized pediatric thymic tumors. Surgeons aim to remove the tumor entirely while preserving surrounding healthy tissue.

b. Radiation Therapy: Radiation therapy may be recommended postoperatively or for unresectable or recurrent tumors to target any residual cancer cells.

c. Chemotherapy: Chemotherapy may be used in cases of advanced or metastatic pediatric thymic tumors, typically employing combinations of chemotherapy agents.

d. Targeted Therapy: In some instances, targeted therapies that specifically target certain molecular markers may be considered, especially for thymic carcinomas.

e. Immunotherapy: Immunotherapy, such as immune checkpoint inhibitors, has shown promise in the treatment of thymic tumors in some cases.

f. Supportive Care: Supportive care interventions, including pain management, nutrition support, and psychosocial support, are essential components of comprehensive pediatric thymic tumor care.

7. Prognosis:

The prognosis for pediatric thymic tumors varies depending on factors such as the tumor subtype, stage, and the success of surgical resection. Thymomas generally have a more favorable prognosis compared to thymic carcinomas, which tend to be more aggressive. Long-term follow-up is essential to monitor for recurrence and late effects of treatment.

8. Challenges and Future Directions:

a. Rarity: The rarity of pediatric thymic tumors poses challenges in terms of diagnosis, treatment guidelines, and research efforts.

b. Late Effects: Understanding and managing the late effects of treatment in pediatric patients is an evolving area of research and clinical care.

c. Survivorship Care: The development of survivorship care plans tailored to pediatric thymic tumor survivors is crucial to address their long-term health needs.

d. Molecular Characterization: Advancements in molecular characterization of thymic tumors may lead to more targeted treatment approaches.

e. International Collaboration: Given the rarity of pediatric thymic tumors, international collaboration and data sharing are vital to advancing research and improving outcomes.

9. Conclusion:

Pediatric thymic tumors, although exceptionally rare, present a unique set of challenges in terms of diagnosis, treatment, and survivorship care. While these tumors share histological similarities with their adult counterparts, their distinct epidemiology and characteristics necessitate specialized approaches to diagnosis and treatment. Ongoing research and collaboration within the medical community are essential to further our understanding of pediatric thymic tumors and improve outcomes for affected children and adolescents.

7.2 Diagnostic Challenges in Pediatric Thymic Tumors

Diagnosing pediatric thymic tumors presents a complex set of challenges due to the rarity of these malignancies and their unique characteristics in children and adolescents. This section explores the diagnostic challenges encountered in pediatric cases of thymic tumors, including issues related to clinical presentation, imaging, histopathology, and the need for a multidisciplinary approach.

1. Rarity and Lack of Awareness:

One of the primary challenges in diagnosing pediatric thymic tumors is their extreme rarity. These tumors account for a minuscule fraction of all pediatric cancers, making them unfamiliar to many healthcare professionals. As a result, there may be a lack of awareness among clinicians regarding the possibility of a thymic tumor when evaluating pediatric patients with mediastinal masses or related symptoms. This lack of awareness can lead to delayed diagnosis and treatment.

2. Nonspecific Clinical Presentation:

Pediatric thymic tumors often present with nonspecific symptoms, which can mimic other more common childhood conditions. These symptoms may include:

- Chest pain
- Cough
- Shortness of breath
- Recurrent respiratory infections
- Fatigue
- Myasthenia Gravis (in rare cases)

Given the overlap of these symptoms with various respiratory and cardiac issues, healthcare providers may initially consider more common diagnoses, leading to a delay in the suspicion and investigation of thymic tumors.

3. Diagnostic Imaging Challenges:

a. Radiological Evaluation: Imaging plays a crucial role in diagnosing pediatric thymic tumors. However, there are challenges associated with radiological evaluation:

- **Location Variability:** Unlike adult thymic tumors, which typically occur in the anterior mediastinum, pediatric thymic tumors can manifest in various mediastinal locations. This variability can make their detection and characterization challenging.
- **Mimicry of Other Conditions:** Thymic tumors may appear similar to other mediastinal masses on imaging, such as lymphomas or neurogenic tumors, further complicating the diagnostic process.
- **Size Variation:** The size of thymic tumors in children can vary significantly, from small lesions to large masses. Smaller tumors may be more challenging to detect on imaging.

b. Role of Contrast Enhancement: The use of contrast-enhanced imaging, such as contrast-enhanced CT scans or MRI, can help differentiate thymic tumors from other mediastinal masses. However, the need for sedation or anesthesia in pediatric patients during MRI scans adds an additional layer of complexity.

c. Radiation Exposure: Minimizing radiation exposure is a priority in pediatric patients. Therefore, using imaging modalities with the lowest possible radiation dose is essential, especially when repeated imaging is necessary for monitoring.

4. Histopathological Complexity:

a. Diverse Histological Subtypes: Thymic tumors encompass a range of histological subtypes, each with distinct characteristics. This diversity can complicate the histopathological diagnosis. Pediatric thymic tumors may include thymomas, thymic carcinomas, and neuroendocrine tumors, among others.

b. Needle Biopsy Limitations: Obtaining a tissue sample for histopathological evaluation often requires a biopsy procedure. In some cases, a needle biopsy may yield insufficient tissue for a definitive diagnosis due to the tumor's location or size. Surgical biopsy may be necessary, which carries inherent risks and requires careful consideration in pediatric patients.

c. Differential Diagnosis: Distinguishing between thymic tumors and other mediastinal lesions, such as lymphomas, germ cell tumors, or neurogenic tumors, is critical for appropriate treatment planning. The histopathological examination plays a central role in making this distinction.

5. Importance of Multidisciplinary Evaluation:

Given the complexity and rarity of pediatric thymic tumors, a multidisciplinary approach is essential. This involves collaboration between various specialists, including pediatric oncologists, pediatric surgeons, radiologists, pathologists, and other relevant healthcare professionals.

a. Pediatric Oncologists: Pediatric oncologists play a central role in the diagnostic process, coordinating evaluations and guiding the treatment plan based on histopathological findings and staging.

b. Pediatric Surgeons: Surgical biopsy or resection is often necessary for diagnosis and treatment. Pediatric surgeons have expertise in performing procedures while minimizing risks in pediatric patients.

c. Radiologists: Radiologists aid in interpreting imaging studies, identifying the location, size, and characteristics of thymic tumors, and distinguishing them from other mediastinal masses.

d. Pathologists: Pathologists provide crucial information through histopathological examination, including the tumor's subtype and grade. Their expertise is vital for guiding treatment decisions.

e. Anesthesiologists: Pediatric patients may require anesthesia for imaging studies or surgical procedures. Anesthesiologists specializing in pediatric care ensure the safety and comfort of young patients during these procedures.

6. Myasthenia Gravis Considerations:

In rare cases, pediatric thymic tumors may be associated with Myasthenia Gravis (MG), an autoimmune neuromuscular disorder. MG can complicate the diagnostic process because its symptoms, such as muscle weakness and difficulty swallowing or breathing, may overshadow other tumor-related symptoms. Identifying MG and its relationship to the thymic tumor is crucial, as it can impact treatment decisions.

7. Challenges in Myasthenia Gravis Testing:

Diagnosing MG in pediatric patients can be challenging, as the disease may present differently than in adults. Specialized testing, such as acetylcholine receptor antibody assays and repetitive nerve stimulation studies, may be required for diagnosis. These tests can be technically demanding and may not be readily available at all healthcare centers.

8. Future Directions and Research:

Addressing the diagnostic challenges associated with

pediatric thymic tumors requires ongoing research and awareness-building efforts:

a. **Clinical Awareness:** Increasing awareness among pediatric healthcare providers about the possibility of thymic tumors in patients with mediastinal masses or related symptoms is essential for early detection.

b. **Research on Imaging Modalities:** Advancements in imaging technology, such as lower-dose CT scans and advanced MRI techniques, can improve the accuracy of diagnosis while minimizing radiation exposure.

c. **Collaboration and Data Sharing:** Collaboration among healthcare institutions and data sharing efforts can enhance our understanding of pediatric thymic tumors and facilitate the development of standardized diagnostic guidelines.

d. **Advances in MG Diagnosis:** Research into more efficient and accessible methods for diagnosing MG in pediatric patients can expedite the identification of this association in thymic tumor cases.

9. Conclusion:

Diagnosing pediatric thymic tumors is a complex process due to their rarity, nonspecific clinical presentation, radiological challenges, and the need for histopathological evaluation. A multidisciplinary approach involving pediatric oncologists, surgeons, radiologists, pathologists, and other specialists is crucial for accurate diagnosis and timely initiation of treatment. Ongoing research, clinical awareness, and advances in diagnostic techniques hold the promise of improving the diagnostic process and ultimately the outcomes for pediatric patients with thymic tumors.

7.3 Pediatric-Specific Treatment Approaches for Thymic

Tumors

Treating thymic tumors in pediatric patients requires a specialized approach tailored to the unique characteristics and challenges of this population. This section explores the distinct treatment modalities and considerations specific to pediatric thymic tumors, including surgical interventions, radiation therapy, chemotherapy, targeted therapy, and the importance of comprehensive care.

1. Multidisciplinary Approach:

The treatment of pediatric thymic tumors necessitates a multidisciplinary team consisting of pediatric oncologists, pediatric surgeons, radiation oncologists, pathologists, and supportive care specialists. The collaboration of these experts ensures that each aspect of a child's care is meticulously planned and executed.

2. Surgical Management:

Surgery is often the primary treatment modality for pediatric thymic tumors, aiming for complete tumor resection while preserving surrounding healthy tissue. Several surgical approaches may be considered:

a. Complete Resection: The primary goal of surgery is to achieve complete resection, which may involve removing the thymic tumor along with surrounding tissue, including the thymus itself. This approach is associated with the best outcomes, particularly for thymomas.

b. Minimally Invasive Surgery: Minimally invasive techniques, such as video-assisted thoracoscopic surgery (VATS), are preferred when feasible, as they result in shorter recovery times and reduced postoperative pain.

c. Sternotomy: In some cases, an open sternotomy may be

necessary for complete tumor removal, especially for larger tumors or those with extensive invasion.

d. Preservation of Adjacent Structures: Pediatric surgeons take special care to preserve nearby structures, such as blood vessels, nerves, and the pericardium, to minimize postoperative complications and long-term morbidity.

e. Assessment of Myasthenia Gravis: In cases associated with Myasthenia Gravis (MG), surgeons may also perform a thymectomy to treat the autoimmune disorder, even if the tumor is benign.

3. Radiation Therapy:

Radiation therapy may be employed in the treatment of pediatric thymic tumors, particularly for unresectable tumors or those with incomplete resection. However, radiation therapy in pediatric patients requires careful consideration due to their unique vulnerabilities:

a. Age-Appropriate Techniques: Pediatric radiation oncologists use age-appropriate techniques to minimize radiation exposure to healthy tissues and organs, ensuring minimal long-term effects.

b. Anesthesia: Young children may require anesthesia during radiation therapy to ensure they remain still and comfortable during the treatment.

c. Late Effects: Efforts are made to reduce the risk of late effects, such as radiation-induced secondary malignancies, by using the lowest effective dose and employing advanced radiation delivery methods.

d. Targeted Radiation: Precise radiation targeting techniques, such as intensity-modulated radiation therapy (IMRT) or proton therapy, can help spare nearby critical structures while effectively treating the tumor.

4. Chemotherapy:

Chemotherapy may be considered for pediatric thymic tumors, especially in cases where the tumor is unresectable, has spread to distant sites (metastasis), or is of a more aggressive histological subtype. Key considerations for pediatric thymic tumor chemotherapy include:

a. Combination Regimens: Chemotherapy regimens typically involve combinations of drugs, such as cisplatin, etoposide, and cyclophosphamide, tailored to the specific tumor and patient.

b. Adjuvant or Neoadjuvant Therapy: Chemotherapy may be administered before or after surgery to shrink the tumor, improve resectability, or reduce the risk of recurrence.

c. Side Effect Management: Managing chemotherapy-related side effects, such as nausea, fatigue, and myelosuppression, is crucial in pediatric patients. Supportive care measures are essential to minimize treatment-related discomfort.

d. Long-Term Monitoring: Pediatric patients receiving chemotherapy require long-term monitoring for potential late effects and complications, including cardiac, renal, or hepatic toxicity.

5. Targeted Therapy:

While not yet a standard treatment for pediatric thymic tumors, targeted therapy is an area of ongoing research and development. Targeted therapies aim to inhibit specific molecular pathways or genetic alterations associated with the tumor, potentially offering more precise and less toxic treatments for children with thymic tumors.

a. Genetic and Molecular Characterization: Understanding the genetic and molecular characteristics of pediatric thymic tumors is essential for identifying potential targets for therapy.

b. Clinical Trials: Pediatric patients may have access to clinical trials exploring targeted therapies as part of their treatment options. These trials can provide innovative and promising treatment strategies.

6. Immunotherapy:

Immunotherapy, particularly immune checkpoint inhibitors, has shown promise in treating thymic tumors in some cases. Immunotherapy works by enhancing the body's immune response against cancer cells. Key considerations for immunotherapy in pediatric thymic tumors include:

a. Patient Selection: Identifying patients who may benefit from immunotherapy based on tumor characteristics, such as the presence of specific immune markers.

b. Immune-Related Adverse Events: Monitoring for and managing immune-related adverse events is crucial in pediatric patients receiving immunotherapy, as these events can affect various organ systems.

c. Clinical Trials: Immunotherapy approaches for pediatric thymic tumors are actively studied in clinical trials, offering potential treatment options beyond conventional therapies.

7. Supportive Care and Survivorship:

Comprehensive care for pediatric thymic tumor patients extends beyond medical treatments and includes holistic support:

a. Psychosocial Support: Pediatric patients and their families may benefit from psychological counseling, support groups, and resources to address the emotional and social challenges of cancer diagnosis and treatment.

b. Pain and Symptom Management: Effective pain and symptom management strategies are essential to enhance the quality of life for pediatric patients undergoing treatment.

c. Nutrition Support: Nutritional assessment and support are crucial, especially if treatment-related side effects impact a child's ability to eat or maintain a healthy weight.

d. Long-Term Monitoring: Pediatric patients require long-term follow-up to monitor for late effects of treatment, assess for recurrence, and address any ongoing health needs.

e. Survivorship Care Plans: Developing survivorship care plans that outline follow-up schedules, potential late effects, and recommended screenings is essential for ensuring the ongoing well-being of pediatric thymic tumor survivors.

8. Future Directions and Research:

Advancements in pediatric thymic tumor treatment continue to evolve. Future directions in research and clinical care include:

a. Molecular Profiling: Further understanding the genetic and molecular characteristics of pediatric thymic tumors to identify potential targets for targeted therapy.

b. Immunotherapy Research: Ongoing investigations into the use of immunotherapy and immune checkpoint inhibitors in pediatric thymic tumors.

c. Survivorship Research: Expanding knowledge of long-term survivorship needs and late effects in pediatric thymic tumor patients.

d. Clinical Trials: Continued participation in clinical trials that explore innovative treatment approaches for pediatric thymic tumors.

9. Conclusion:

Treating pediatric thymic tumors requires a pediatric-specific, multidisciplinary approach that considers the unique characteristics of these rare malignancies and the vulnerabilities of young patients. Surgery remains a primary treatment modality, often combined with radiation therapy, chemotherapy, targeted therapy, or immunotherapy based on the individual case. Comprehensive care, including psychosocial support, pain management, nutrition support, and long-term monitoring, is essential for the well-being of pediatric thymic tumor patients. Ongoing research and clinical trials hold the promise of advancing treatment options and improving outcomes for this rare pediatric population.

7.4 Long-Term Effects and Follow-Up in Pediatric Patients with Thymic Tumors

While successful treatment of thymic tumors in pediatric patients is a significant achievement, it's essential to recognize that these young survivors may face unique long-term effects and challenges. This section explores the potential late effects of treatment, the importance of comprehensive follow-up care, and the development of survivorship care plans tailored to the needs of pediatric thymic tumor survivors.

1. Understanding Long-Term Effects:

Long-term effects, also known as late effects, are health issues that may arise months or even years after completing treatment for thymic tumors. These late effects can result from the tumor itself, the treatments received, or a combination of both. Pediatric patients who have battled thymic tumors are at risk for specific late effects due to their young age and the nature of treatment. These late effects can affect various aspects of their physical, emotional, and social well-being.

2. Potential Late Effects:

a. Cardiac Complications: Radiation therapy and certain chemotherapy agents may increase the risk of cardiovascular issues in pediatric thymic tumor survivors. Late effects can include cardiomyopathy, valvular heart disease, and coronary artery disease. Monitoring cardiac health through regular assessments is crucial.

b. Pulmonary Concerns: The chest area, which includes the lungs, may have been exposed to radiation during treatment. Late pulmonary effects can include radiation-induced lung fibrosis or scarring, which may lead to breathing difficulties. Lung function tests and imaging are essential for monitoring lung health.

c. Endocrine Disorders: Radiation therapy can affect the endocrine system, potentially leading to hormonal imbalances and disorders, such as hypothyroidism or growth hormone deficiency. Regular endocrine assessments and hormone replacement therapy, when necessary, are part of follow-up care.

d. Secondary Malignancies: Pediatric patients treated for thymic tumors may have an increased risk of developing secondary malignancies due to radiation exposure. Surveillance through cancer screening protocols is essential for early detection and intervention.

e. Cognitive and Developmental Issues: Pediatric patients may experience cognitive or developmental delays or deficits, especially if treatments affect the central nervous system. Neuropsychological assessments can help identify and address these issues.

f. Emotional and Psychosocial Challenges: Pediatric thymic tumor survivors may face emotional and psychosocial challenges related to their cancer journey, including anxiety, depression, or post-traumatic stress. Access to counseling and support services is vital for their well-being.

g. Educational and Social Impact: Long-term treatment may disrupt a child's education and social development. Educational support, including tutoring and special accommodations, can help survivors catch up academically and socially.

h. Fertility Concerns: Some treatments for thymic tumors may impact fertility in the long term. Fertility preservation discussions and options should be available for patients approaching adolescence.

i. Myasthenia Gravis: If Myasthenia Gravis (MG) was associated with the thymic tumor, its management and potential recurrence should be monitored.

3. Survivorship Care Plans:

To address the long-term health needs of pediatric thymic tumor survivors comprehensively, healthcare providers develop survivorship care plans (SCPs). These plans are tailored to the individual survivor's medical history, treatments received, and potential late effects. Key components of SCPs include:

a. Follow-Up Schedule: SCPs outline a schedule for follow-up appointments and screenings to monitor for potential late effects or recurrence. These schedules may include regular visits to pediatric oncologists, cardiologists, endocrinologists, and other specialists as needed.

b. Imaging and Testing: Specific tests and imaging studies are recommended based on the survivor's treatment history. For example, echocardiograms or pulmonary function tests may be part of the routine assessment.

c. Health Promotion: SCPs emphasize the importance of a healthy lifestyle, including nutrition, physical activity, and smoking cessation, to minimize the risk of late effects and promote overall well-being.

d. Education: Providing survivors and their families with information about potential late effects, symptoms to watch for, and coping strategies is essential for informed decision-making and proactive health management.

e. Psychosocial Support: Emotional and psychosocial support resources are integrated into SCPs to address survivors' mental health needs and facilitate adjustment to life after cancer treatment.

f. Reproductive Health: For survivors approaching adolescence, discussions about fertility preservation options should be included in SCPs to ensure informed choices about future family planning.

4. Survivorship Clinics:

Many pediatric oncology centers have established survivorship clinics or programs that specialize in long-term follow-up care. These clinics offer a centralized approach to monitoring survivors' health, addressing late effects, and providing ongoing support. Pediatric oncologists and other specialists collaborate within these clinics to deliver comprehensive care.

5. Transitioning to Adult Care:

As pediatric thymic tumor survivors reach adulthood, they face the transition from pediatric to adult healthcare services.

This transition can be challenging, as adult healthcare systems may differ in structure and approach. To facilitate a smooth transition, healthcare providers often work with adolescent and young adult (AYA) oncology programs that are equipped to address the unique needs of this age group.

6. Importance of Patient and Family Engagement:

Engaging pediatric thymic tumor survivors and their families in their care is crucial for successful long-term management. Open communication, shared decision-making, and empowerment of survivors to advocate for their health contribute to improved outcomes.

7. Research and Advancements:

Ongoing research in the field of pediatric thymic tumors aims to further understand the long-term effects of treatment and develop strategies to mitigate these effects. Clinical trials exploring innovative treatments and follow-up care approaches continue to expand the knowledge base and improve outcomes for survivors.

8. Conclusion:

Pediatric thymic tumor survivors deserve comprehensive, lifelong care that addresses their unique long-term health needs and potential late effects. Survivorship care plans, developed in collaboration with healthcare providers, play a pivotal role in monitoring survivors' health, addressing late effects, and promoting overall well-being. Engaging survivors and their families in their care, ensuring access to support services, and staying informed about research advancements are essential components of caring for these young survivors as they embark on their journey beyond cancer.

7.5 Future Directions in Pediatric Thymic Tumor Research

The field of pediatric thymic tumor research has made significant strides in recent years, but many questions remain unanswered, and challenges persist. As we look to the future, it is imperative to outline key areas of research and innovation that hold promise for advancing our understanding and improving outcomes for young patients with thymic tumors. This section explores the exciting and evolving landscape of research in pediatric thymic tumors.

1. Genetic and Molecular Profiling:

One of the most promising directions in pediatric thymic tumor research is the extensive genetic and molecular characterization of these rare tumors. Understanding the underlying genetic alterations and molecular pathways driving thymic tumor development is essential for several reasons:

a. Targeted Therapies: Identifying specific genetic mutations or molecular markers associated with thymic tumors can pave the way for targeted therapies. These therapies aim to disrupt or inhibit the molecular pathways driving tumor growth, potentially leading to more effective and less toxic treatments.

b. Personalized Medicine: Genetic and molecular profiling can enable the development of personalized treatment plans tailored to each patient's unique tumor characteristics. This approach increases the likelihood of successful outcomes by selecting treatments that are most likely to be effective.

c. Biomarker Discovery: Research efforts may uncover novel biomarkers that can aid in early diagnosis, prognosis prediction, and treatment response monitoring in pediatric thymic tumors.

d. Genomic Research Consortia: Collaboration among research institutions and international genomic consortia can accelerate progress in this area, pooling data and expertise to unravel the genetic complexities of pediatric thymic tumors.

2. Immunotherapy Advancements:

Immunotherapy, particularly immune checkpoint inhibitors, has shown promise in the treatment of thymic tumors in some cases. Future research directions in immunotherapy for pediatric thymic tumors include:

a. Patient Stratification: Identifying the subset of pediatric thymic tumor patients most likely to benefit from immunotherapy based on their tumor's immunological characteristics and immune marker expression.

b. Combination Therapies: Exploring the potential of combining immunotherapy with other treatment modalities, such as targeted therapy or chemotherapy, to enhance treatment responses and durability.

c. Immune-Related Adverse Events: Investigating strategies to mitigate and manage immune-related adverse events associated with immunotherapy, especially in the pediatric population.

d. Biomarkers of Response: Identifying reliable biomarkers that predict immunotherapy response and resistance in pediatric thymic tumor patients.

e. Clinical Trials: Conducting clinical trials focused on immunotherapy approaches tailored to the specific needs of pediatric patients, including age-appropriate dosing and monitoring.

3. Pediatric-Specific Clinical Trials:

Clinical trials are instrumental in advancing treatment options for pediatric thymic tumor patients. Future directions in clinical research include:

a. Targeted Pediatric Trials: Designing clinical trials specifically for pediatric thymic tumor patients, considering their unique needs, vulnerabilities, and tumor characteristics.

b. Combination Therapies: Investigating combination therapies that incorporate surgery, radiation therapy, chemotherapy, targeted therapy, and immunotherapy to optimize treatment outcomes.

c. Long-Term Follow-Up: Implementing long-term follow-up protocols in clinical trials to monitor late effects, survivorship issues, and treatment durability.

d. Quality of Life Assessments: Integrating assessments of quality of life, psychosocial well-being, and developmental outcomes as important endpoints in clinical trials.

e. Pediatric Enrollment: Encouraging greater enrollment of pediatric patients in clinical trials through awareness campaigns and improved access to cutting-edge treatments.

4. Early Detection and Screening:

Early detection of pediatric thymic tumors is crucial for improving outcomes. Future research directions in this area include:

a. Biomarker Discovery: Investigating blood-based biomarkers or imaging techniques that can facilitate early detection and risk stratification.

b. Genetic Screening: Evaluating the feasibility and effectiveness of genetic screening for pediatric thymic tumor predisposition in high-risk populations or families with a history of thymic tumors.

c. Artificial Intelligence (AI): Leveraging AI and machine learning algorithms to analyze medical imaging data for early detection and risk prediction.

d. Screening Guidelines: Developing evidence-based screening guidelines for pediatric thymic tumors, particularly in high-risk populations.

5. Survivorship Research:

Research focused on the long-term outcomes and quality of life of pediatric thymic tumor survivors is essential. Future directions in survivorship research include:

a. Late Effects Studies: Conducting comprehensive studies to understand the prevalence and impact of late effects in pediatric survivors, with a focus on cardiac, pulmonary, endocrine, cognitive, and psychosocial aspects.

b. Survivorship Care Models: Developing survivorship care models that cater to the unique needs of pediatric thymic tumor survivors, addressing physical, emotional, educational, and social aspects of their lives.

c. Transition to Adult Care: Investigating strategies and interventions that facilitate a smooth transition from pediatric to adult healthcare services for survivors.

d. Fertility Preservation: Advancing research in fertility preservation options for adolescents and young adults who may face fertility challenges due to treatment.

6. International Collaborations:

Collaboration among research institutions, healthcare providers, and advocacy groups on a global scale is crucial for advancing pediatric thymic tumor research. Future directions in international collaboration include:

a. Data Sharing: Promoting data sharing and collaboration across borders to facilitate larger-scale studies and increase the statistical power of research findings.

b. Standardized Protocols: Developing and implementing standardized protocols for the diagnosis, treatment, and follow-up of pediatric thymic tumors to ensure consistency and comparability of research outcomes.

c. Rare Disease Networks: Engaging with international rare disease networks to raise awareness, share best practices, and support research efforts in pediatric thymic tumors.

7. Patient and Family Engagement:

Involving patients and their families in the research process is vital. Future directions include:

a. Patient Advocacy: Encouraging and supporting patient and family advocacy groups to raise awareness, fund research, and actively participate in research initiatives.

b. Patient-Reported Outcomes: Incorporating patient-reported outcomes and perspectives into research design, ensuring that research questions and outcomes align with the priorities of those affected by thymic tumors.

c. Shared Decision-Making: Promoting shared decision-making between healthcare providers, researchers, and patients and their families to ensure that research efforts address the most pressing needs.

8. Public Awareness and Education:

Raising public awareness about pediatric thymic tumors is essential for early detection, funding, and support. Future directions include:

a. Education Campaigns: Launching educational campaigns to inform healthcare providers, schools, and the public about the signs and symptoms of thymic tumors and the importance of early diagnosis.

b. Research Advocacy: Engaging celebrities, philanthropists, and public figures in research advocacy efforts to increase funding and support for pediatric thymic tumor research.

c. Online Resources: Expanding the availability of online resources, support groups, and educational materials for patients, families, and healthcare providers.

9. Conclusion:

The future of pediatric thymic tumor research is filled with promise, driven by advances in genetics, immunotherapy, clinical trials, early detection, survivorship care, international collaborations, patient engagement, and public awareness efforts. By investing in these directions and maintaining a collective commitment to improving the lives of young patients with thymic tumors, we can look forward to a future where better treatments, earlier diagnoses, and enhanced support lead to improved outcomes and increased hope for pediatric thymic tumor patients and their families.

7.6 Psychosocial and Family Support for Pediatric Patients with Thymic Tumors

The journey of pediatric patients diagnosed with thymic tumors is not solely medical; it also encompasses profound emotional, psychological, and social aspects that influence both the child and their family. This section explores the critical role of psychosocial support and the importance of a strong support network for pediatric patients facing thymic tumors.

1. The Psychosocial Impact of Pediatric Thymic Tumors:

The diagnosis of a thymic tumor in a child can be

an overwhelming and emotionally charged experience for both the young patient and their family. Understanding the psychosocial impact is essential for providing effective support:

a. Emotional Distress: Children may experience a range of emotions, including fear, anxiety, sadness, and anger, in response to their diagnosis and treatment. The uncertainty of the disease and the disruption to their normal lives can contribute to emotional distress.

b. Impact on Family: The entire family unit is affected when a child is diagnosed with a thymic tumor. Parents and siblings may experience stress, guilt, and anxiety. The dynamics within the family may change, with roles shifting to accommodate the demands of the illness.

c. Social Isolation: Pediatric patients with thymic tumors may feel socially isolated due to their illness. They may miss school, extracurricular activities, and social events, which can lead to feelings of loneliness and isolation.

d. Developmental Challenges: The experience of battling a thymic tumor can disrupt a child's normal developmental milestones, including educational progress, friendships, and identity formation.

e. Traumatic Stress: In some cases, the diagnosis and treatment of a thymic tumor can be traumatic, leading to post-traumatic stress symptoms that require specialized support.

2. The Role of Psychosocial Support:

Psychosocial support plays a pivotal role in addressing the emotional, psychological, and social needs of pediatric patients with thymic tumors and their families:

a. Emotional Support: Providing a safe space for children to express their feelings, concerns, and fears is crucial. Psychosocial professionals, such as child life specialists, psychologists, and social workers, can offer emotional support through individual and group counseling sessions.

b. Education and Information: Offering age-appropriate information and education about the disease, treatment, and potential side effects helps children and their families feel more in control and less anxious.

c. Coping Strategies: Teaching coping strategies and relaxation techniques, such as mindfulness and deep breathing exercises, empowers pediatric patients to manage stress and anxiety.

d. Peer Support: Connecting pediatric patients with thymic tumors with peers who have gone through similar experiences can alleviate feelings of isolation and provide a sense of belonging.

e. Sibling Support: Recognizing the impact of a thymic tumor diagnosis on siblings and offering sibling support programs can help siblings navigate their emotions and concerns.

f. Parental Support: Parents require substantial support, too. Parent support groups, counseling, and resources can help them manage their own stress, make informed decisions, and effectively support their child.

g. School and Educational Support: Collaborating with schools to provide educational support and accommodations during treatment and recovery ensures that children can maintain their academic progress and feel connected to their peers.

3. Family-Centered Care:

Family-centered care is a holistic approach that recognizes

the importance of involving the entire family in the child's healthcare journey:

a. **Shared Decision-Making:** Including parents and, when age-appropriate, the pediatric patient in treatment decisions fosters a sense of partnership and empowerment.

b. **Comprehensive Assessment:** Healthcare providers assess not only the child's physical health but also their emotional and psychosocial well-being. This approach helps identify specific support needs.

c. **Communication:** Open and transparent communication between healthcare providers, pediatric patients, and their families is critical for building trust and ensuring that everyone is informed about the treatment plan and progress.

d. **Coordination of Care:** Coordinating medical, psychosocial, and educational support services ensures that the child and family receive comprehensive care that addresses their unique needs.

4. Supportive Resources and Programs:

Several resources and programs are available to provide psychosocial support to pediatric patients with thymic tumors and their families:

a. **Child Life Programs:** Child life specialists are trained professionals who help children understand and cope with healthcare experiences through play, preparation, and education. They create a child-friendly environment within the hospital setting.

b. **Psychologists and Social Workers:** These professionals offer individual and family counseling, emotional support, and coping strategies to help pediatric patients and their families navigate the challenges of thymic tumors.

c. Support Groups: Support groups bring together pediatric patients and families facing similar challenges. These groups provide a platform for sharing experiences, gaining insights, and building a sense of community.

d. Educational Liaisons: Educational liaisons work with schools to ensure that pediatric patients receive the necessary support to continue their education during treatment and recovery.

e. Art and Music Therapy: Creative therapies, such as art and music therapy, offer children alternative ways to express themselves and cope with the emotional impact of thymic tumors.

f. Play and Recreation Programs: These programs provide opportunities for children to engage in age-appropriate play and recreational activities, promoting normalcy and fun during their hospital stay.

5. Transitioning to Survivorship:

As pediatric patients with thymic tumors transition to survivorship, their psychosocial needs continue to evolve:

a. Survivorship Clinics: Survivorship clinics offer long-term follow-up care that addresses not only medical needs but also psychosocial and educational aspects of survivorship.

b. Educational and Vocational Support: Adolescent and young adult survivors may require support in pursuing their educational and vocational goals, which can be affected by their cancer experience.

c. Coping with Survivorship Challenges: Survivors may encounter challenges related to body image, relationships, and psychosocial well-being. Psychosocial support remains crucial during this phase.

d. Fertility Counseling: For survivors approaching adolescence, discussions about fertility preservation options should be available to ensure informed choices about future family planning.

6. The Role of Advocacy:

Advocacy organizations and individuals play a vital role in raising awareness about the psychosocial needs of pediatric patients with thymic tumors:

a. Fundraising and Awareness Campaigns: Advocacy efforts can raise funds for psychosocial support programs and campaigns to increase awareness about the unique challenges faced by pediatric thymic tumor patients and their families.

b. Legislative Advocacy: Advocacy organizations can lobby for policies and legislation that support psychosocial care and resources for pediatric cancer patients.

c. Parent and Survivor Advocacy: Parents and survivors can become advocates for the psychosocial well-being of pediatric patients, sharing their experiences and advocating for improved support services.

7. Conclusion:

Psychosocial support is an integral component of the care provided to pediatric patients with thymic tumors and their families. Recognizing the emotional and psychosocial impact of a thymic tumor diagnosis and addressing the unique needs of young patients and their families are essential for improving overall well-being and enhancing the quality of life during and after treatment. By offering a comprehensive support network that includes emotional counseling, educational assistance, sibling support, and family-centered care, healthcare providers and advocacy organizations can ensure that pediatric patients and their families receive the holistic care they need to navigate this challenging journey with resilience and hope.

CHAPTER 8: HOLISTIC HEALTH AND WELL-BEING

8.1 Integrative Medicine and Thymic Tumor Patients: Holistic Approaches to Support Healing

Integrative medicine is an approach to healthcare that combines conventional medical treatments with complementary and alternative therapies to address the physical, emotional, and psychosocial aspects of a patient's well-being. For pediatric and adult patients diagnosed with thymic tumors, integrative medicine offers a holistic framework to support healing, improve quality of life, and enhance the overall healthcare experience. In this section, we explore the principles of integrative medicine and its application in the care of thymic tumor patients.

1. Understanding Integrative Medicine:

Integrative medicine represents a shift in the healthcare paradigm, acknowledging that optimal health and healing encompass more than just the absence of disease. Key principles of integrative medicine include:

a. Patient-Centered Care: Integrative medicine places the patient at the center of the healthcare journey, emphasizing a collaborative and individualized approach to care.

b. Holistic Approach: It recognizes that health is influenced by physical, emotional, social, and environmental factors, and that all aspects of a patient's life should be considered in their care.

c. Evidence-Based Practice: Integrative medicine incorporates evidence-based complementary therapies and treatments that have demonstrated safety and efficacy.

d. Prevention and Wellness: A primary focus is on preventive measures and promoting overall wellness to reduce the risk of recurrence and improve long-term outcomes.

e. Open Communication: Effective communication and partnership between healthcare providers, patients, and their families are emphasized, ensuring that treatment decisions align with patients' values and preferences.

2. Complementary and Alternative Therapies:

Integrative medicine encompasses a wide range of complementary and alternative therapies that can be integrated into the care of thymic tumor patients. These therapies aim to enhance the body's natural healing abilities, manage symptoms, and improve quality of life. Some examples include:

a. Mind-Body Practices: Techniques such as mindfulness meditation, yoga, and tai chi promote relaxation, reduce stress, and improve emotional well-being.

b. Acupuncture and Acupressure: These therapies can help manage pain, nausea, and other treatment-related side effects.

c. Nutrition and Dietary Counseling: Guidance on proper nutrition can support overall health and energy levels during treatment and recovery.

d. Herbal Medicine and Supplements: Certain herbs and supplements may have potential benefits for symptom management and immune support.

e. Massage and Bodywork: Massage therapy can relieve muscle tension, reduce anxiety, and improve circulation.

f. Art and Music Therapy: These creative therapies provide an outlet for expression, reduce stress, and improve mood.

g. Energy Therapies: Practices like Reiki and Healing Touch focus on balancing the body's energy systems to promote healing.

3. Pain and Symptom Management:

Pain and symptom management are central to the integrative care of thymic tumor patients. Integrative approaches can:

a. Reduce Pain: Complementary therapies such as acupuncture, massage, and relaxation techniques can help alleviate pain, allowing for lower doses of pain medications.

b. Manage Treatment Side Effects: Integrative therapies can address common side effects of thymic tumor treatments, such as nausea, fatigue, and neuropathy.

c. Improve Sleep: Mind-body practices and relaxation techniques can promote better sleep patterns, which are essential for healing.

d. Enhance Emotional Well-Being: Integrative medicine offers tools and strategies to manage stress, anxiety, and depression that often accompany a cancer diagnosis and treatment.

4. Nutritional Support:

Nutrition plays a critical role in the overall health and well-being of thymic tumor patients. Integrative medicine can provide guidance on:

a. Balanced Diets: Recommendations for a balanced and nourishing diet that supports the immune system and overall health during and after treatment.

b. Managing Nutritional Challenges: Addressing nutritional challenges such as loss of appetite, taste changes, and difficulty swallowing that may arise during treatment.

c. Dietary Supplements: Assessing the use of dietary supplements to meet specific nutritional needs or manage side effects.

5. Emotional and Psychosocial Support:

The emotional and psychosocial aspects of cancer care are integral to integrative medicine. Supportive services may include:

a. Counseling: Individual and family counseling to address emotional distress, coping strategies, and communication.

b. Support Groups: Participation in support groups where patients and families can connect with others facing similar challenges.

c. Mindfulness and Stress Reduction: Techniques such as mindfulness meditation and relaxation exercises to reduce stress and improve emotional well-being.

d. Expressive Therapies: Art and music therapy as outlets for self-expression and emotional processing.

6. Survivorship and Quality of Life:

Integrative medicine extends its benefits beyond the active treatment phase, focusing on survivorship and long-term quality of life:

a. Survivorship Care Plans: Development of survivorship care plans that include recommendations for ongoing integrative care to address late effects and support emotional well-being.

b. Monitoring Late Effects: Continual monitoring for late effects of treatment, including cardiac, pulmonary, and psychosocial aspects, with interventions as needed.

c. Fertility Preservation: Discussions about fertility preservation options for adolescent and young adult patients approaching adulthood.

d. Educational and Vocational Support: Support for adolescents and young adults in pursuing their educational and vocational goals.

e. Coping with Body Image Issues: Addressing issues related to body image and self-esteem that may arise due to the effects of treatment.

7. Collaborative Care:

Integrative medicine is most effective when integrated into a patient's overall care plan. Collaboration between conventional medical practitioners and integrative medicine specialists is crucial:

a. Team-Based Care: A collaborative healthcare team, including oncologists, surgeons, nurses, and integrative medicine practitioners, ensures that patients receive comprehensive care that addresses all aspects of their well-being.

b. Coordinated Approaches: Regular communication and coordination between all healthcare providers ensure that integrative therapies complement rather than contradict conventional treatments.

c. Shared Decision-Making: Patients are actively involved in decisions regarding their integrative care, with healthcare providers offering evidence-based guidance and respecting patients' preferences.

8. Conclusion:

Integrative medicine offers a holistic approach to the care of thymic tumor patients, addressing not only the physical aspects of the disease but also the emotional, psychosocial, and overall well-being of the patient. By incorporating evidence-based complementary therapies, nutrition guidance, pain and symptom management, and emotional support, integrative medicine can enhance the quality of life, improve treatment outcomes, and empower patients to actively participate in their healing journey. Collaborative, patient-centered care that integrates the best of both conventional and complementary medicine is essential for the comprehensive care of thymic tumor patients across the lifespan.

8.2 Nutrition and Dietary Guidelines for Thymic Tumor Patients

Nutrition plays a pivotal role in the overall health and well-being of individuals diagnosed with thymic tumors. Proper nutrition can support the immune system, aid in managing treatment-related side effects, and promote overall vitality. In this section, we will explore nutrition and dietary guidelines specifically tailored to thymic tumor patients, emphasizing the importance of personalized dietary plans and addressing common nutritional challenges that may arise during treatment and recovery.

1. The Significance of Nutrition in Thymic Tumor Care:

Maintaining adequate nutrition is essential for individuals diagnosed with thymic tumors. A well-balanced diet can serve several vital purposes:

a. Immune Support: Proper nutrition provides essential nutrients that support the immune system, helping the body defend against infections and illness.

b. Treatment Tolerance: A healthy diet can improve treatment tolerance and reduce the risk of treatment interruptions by supporting overall strength and vitality.

c. Recovery and Healing: Nutrient-rich foods can aid in the healing process, promoting tissue repair and reducing recovery time.

d. Quality of Life: Good nutrition can enhance the quality of life by managing treatment-related side effects, such as nausea, fatigue, and weight changes.

e. Long-Term Health: Establishing healthy eating habits during and after treatment can contribute to long-term health and reduce the risk of chronic diseases.

2. Personalized Nutrition Plans:

Thymic tumor patients have unique nutritional needs, influenced by factors such as their age, treatment regimen, overall health, and any existing nutritional challenges. Therefore, personalized nutrition plans are essential. Key considerations for tailoring nutrition plans include:

a. Treatment Phase: Nutrition requirements may vary during different phases of treatment, such as surgery, chemotherapy, radiation therapy, or post-treatment recovery.

b. Age and Developmental Stage: Pediatric patients, adolescents, and adults have differing nutritional needs based on their growth and development.

c. Treatment-Related Side Effects: Specific dietary strategies can address common side effects like nausea, taste changes, appetite loss, and swallowing difficulties.

d. Preexisting Conditions: Patients with preexisting conditions, such as diabetes or heart disease, may need specialized dietary plans that take these conditions into account.

e. Cultural and Personal Preferences: Dietary plans should respect cultural and personal food preferences to ensure compliance and enjoyment of meals.

3. Key Components of a Nutritional Plan:

A comprehensive nutritional plan for thymic tumor patients should include the following key components:

a. Balanced Diet: A diet rich in fruits, vegetables, whole grains, lean proteins, and healthy fats provides a wide range of essential nutrients.

b. Adequate Calories: Maintaining a healthy weight and adequate calorie intake is crucial for energy levels and overall well-being.

c. Protein Intake: Protein is essential for tissue repair and immune function. Including lean sources of protein is important.

d. Hydration: Staying well-hydrated is vital, especially during treatment, to prevent dehydration and support bodily functions.

e. Nutrient Supplements: Depending on individual needs, healthcare providers may recommend specific nutrient supplements to address deficiencies.

4. Managing Common Nutritional Challenges:

Thymic tumor patients may face several nutritional

challenges during their journey. Addressing these challenges can improve overall nutrition and quality of life:

a. Nausea and Vomiting: Eating smaller, more frequent meals, consuming bland foods, and staying hydrated can help manage nausea and vomiting. Antiemetic medications prescribed by healthcare providers may also be beneficial.

b. Taste Changes: Changes in taste perception can make food less appealing. Experimenting with different flavors and textures and focusing on favorite foods can help improve the dining experience.

c. Loss of Appetite: Strategies such as eating smaller, nutrient-dense meals, drinking high-calorie shakes, and maintaining regular eating schedules can help increase calorie intake.

d. Swallowing Difficulties: Soft or pureed foods, as well as thickened liquids, may be recommended for patients with difficulty swallowing. Speech therapists can provide guidance.

e. Weight Management: Patients may experience weight gain or loss during treatment. Nutritionists can create plans to address these issues, whether through calorie control or nutrient supplementation.

5. Nutritional Considerations for Pediatric Patients:

Pediatric thymic tumor patients have specific nutritional needs that must be addressed to support their growth and development:

a. Adequate Calories: Children need sufficient calories to fuel their growth, especially during active treatment phases.

b. Nutrient Density: Nutrient-dense foods are crucial to ensure that every calorie counts towards meeting the child's nutritional needs.

c. Pediatric Formulas: In some cases, healthcare providers may recommend specialized pediatric formulas to ensure adequate nutrition.

d. Monitoring Growth: Regular monitoring of a child's growth and nutritional status is essential to detect any issues early and adjust the dietary plan accordingly.

e. Family Involvement: Engaging the entire family in meal planning and encouraging a positive food environment can enhance compliance and support the child's nutrition.

6. Long-Term Nutrition and Survivorship:

Nutritional care does not end with the completion of treatment. Long-term nutrition and survivorship considerations include:

a. Monitoring Nutritional Status: Regular check-ups and nutritional assessments help monitor and maintain proper nutrition during survivorship.

b. Healthy Eating Habits: Encouraging lifelong healthy eating habits can reduce the risk of long-term health issues.

c. Fertility and Hormonal Considerations: Adolescent and young adult survivors may require counseling on fertility preservation and hormonal health.

d. Addressing Late Effects: Nutritional plans should consider late effects of treatment, such as cardiac or pulmonary issues, and address them as needed.

e. Educational and Vocational Support: Adolescents and young adults should receive support for pursuing their educational and vocational goals.

7. Conclusion:

Nutrition and dietary guidelines are integral to the care of thymic tumor patients, supporting their immune function, treatment tolerance, recovery, and long-term health. Personalized nutrition plans, addressing common nutritional challenges, and considering age-specific needs are essential components of comprehensive nutritional care. Whether during active treatment, in survivorship, or throughout the lifespan, proper nutrition plays a vital role in enhancing the overall well-being and quality of life of thymic tumor patients. Collaborative efforts between healthcare providers, nutritionists, and patients are key to ensuring that nutritional goals align with treatment objectives and individual preferences.

8.3 Exercise and Physical Rehabilitation for Thymic Tumor Patients

Exercise and physical rehabilitation are often overlooked aspects of cancer care but play a vital role in improving the overall health and well-being of thymic tumor patients. In this section, we will explore the importance of exercise, its potential benefits, and the role of physical rehabilitation in supporting thymic tumor patients throughout their journey.

1. Understanding the Role of Exercise:

Physical activity and exercise are essential components of a holistic approach to cancer care, including thymic tumors. Exercise offers several potential benefits for thymic tumor patients:

a. Improved Physical Function: Regular exercise can enhance physical fitness, strength, and endurance, helping patients better tolerate treatment-related side effects.

b. Enhanced Immune Function: Exercise has been shown to

boost the immune system, potentially aiding the body's ability to fight cancer cells and infections.

c. Reduced Fatigue: Engaging in physical activity can reduce cancer-related fatigue, one of the most common side effects of cancer treatment.

d. Better Psychological Well-being: Exercise can improve mood, reduce anxiety and depression, and enhance overall psychological well-being.

e. Weight Management: For patients experiencing weight changes during treatment, exercise can help maintain a healthy weight or manage weight loss or gain.

f. Enhanced Quality of Life: Regular physical activity can improve overall quality of life by promoting a sense of well-being and normalcy.

2. Tailoring Exercise Plans:

Exercise plans for thymic tumor patients should be individualized, taking into account the patient's age, overall health, treatment phase, and any specific physical limitations. Key considerations for tailoring exercise plans include:

a. Treatment Phase: The exercise regimen may need to be adjusted depending on whether the patient is in the active treatment phase, recovery phase, or long-term survivorship.

b. Age and Developmental Stage: Pediatric, adolescent, and adult patients have different exercise needs based on their growth, development, and physical abilities.

c. Treatment-Related Limitations: Some patients may have physical limitations due to surgery or treatment side effects. Exercise plans must accommodate these limitations.

d. Personal Preferences: The exercise plan should align with the patient's personal interests and preferences to enhance motivation and adherence.

e. Safety Precautions: Safety considerations, such as maintaining proper hydration and avoiding high-risk activities, should be incorporated into the exercise plan.

3. Types of Exercise for Thymic Tumor Patients:

Thymic tumor patients can benefit from a variety of exercise modalities, including:

a. Aerobic Exercise: Activities like walking, cycling, swimming, and dancing can improve cardiovascular fitness, reduce fatigue, and boost mood.

b. Strength Training: Resistance exercises with weights or resistance bands can help build muscle strength and endurance, aiding in physical function.

c. Flexibility and Stretching: Stretching exercises can enhance flexibility, reduce the risk of muscle tightness, and improve overall mobility.

d. Balance and Coordination: Balance exercises can be particularly beneficial for patients who have undergone surgery or experienced balance-related issues.

e. Yoga and Tai Chi: Mind-body practices like yoga and tai chi promote relaxation, improve flexibility, and enhance psychological well-being.

f. Supervised Rehabilitation: Some patients may benefit from supervised rehabilitation programs that are tailored to their specific needs and limitations.

4. Managing Treatment-Related Side Effects:

Exercise can be particularly effective in managing treatment-related side effects commonly experienced by thymic tumor patients:

a. Fatigue: Moderate-intensity exercise has been shown to reduce cancer-related fatigue. Patients can start with short, low-intensity sessions and gradually increase the duration and intensity as tolerated.

b. Muscle Weakness: Strength training exercises can help rebuild muscle strength and combat weakness caused by surgery or treatment.

c. Pain Management: Physical therapy and exercises prescribed by healthcare providers can assist in managing pain and discomfort.

d. Shortness of Breath: Breathing exercises and low-intensity aerobic activities can help improve lung function and reduce shortness of breath.

e. Anxiety and Depression: Exercise has a positive impact on mood and can be used as an adjunct therapy to help manage anxiety and depression.

5. Exercise Safety and Precautions:

Safety is a paramount concern when designing exercise plans for thymic tumor patients:

a. Healthcare Provider Consultation: Before starting any exercise program, patients should consult their healthcare providers to ensure that exercise is safe and appropriate for their individual circumstances.

b. Gradual Progression: Patients should start with low-intensity exercises and gradually increase the intensity and duration as tolerated.

c. Hydration: Staying well-hydrated is essential, especially during exercise, to prevent dehydration.

d. Monitoring: Patients should be encouraged to monitor their physical symptoms during exercise and adjust their activities accordingly.

e. Supervision: Some patients, particularly those with significant limitations, may benefit from supervised exercise programs led by qualified professionals.

6. Rehabilitation and Physical Therapy:

Physical rehabilitation and therapy are crucial components of thymic tumor care, especially for patients who have undergone surgery or experienced physical limitations due to their condition. The role of rehabilitation includes:

a. Preoperative Preparation: For patients undergoing surgery, preoperative physical therapy can optimize physical function and prepare the body for surgery.

b. Postoperative Recovery: Post-surgery rehabilitation focuses on regaining strength, mobility, and function after the procedure.

c. Managing Treatment Effects: Rehabilitation can help patients manage the physical effects of treatment, such as weakness, pain, and reduced mobility.

d. Functional Restoration: Physical therapists work with patients to restore functional abilities, such as walking, balance, and daily activities.

e. Pain Management: Rehabilitation can include techniques for managing treatment-related pain and discomfort.

7. Supportive Care and Survivorship:

Exercise and physical rehabilitation remain important

throughout the survivorship phase of thymic tumor care:

a. **Survivorship Care Plans:** Survivorship care plans may include recommendations for maintaining regular exercise and addressing any late effects of treatment.

b. **Monitoring and Assessments:** Regular monitoring of physical function and assessments by rehabilitation specialists can detect and address issues early.

c. **Long-Term Health:** Engaging in regular exercise contributes to long-term health, reducing the risk of chronic conditions and promoting overall well-being.

d. **Emotional Well-being:** Exercise can continue to support emotional well-being and reduce the risk of anxiety and depression during survivorship.

8. Conclusion:

Exercise and physical rehabilitation are integral components of thymic tumor care, contributing to improved physical function, enhanced quality of life, and better overall well-being. Tailored exercise plans that consider the patient's age, treatment phase, physical limitations, and personal preferences are essential. Rehabilitation plays a vital role in optimizing physical function, managing treatment effects, and supporting survivorship. Collaboration between healthcare providers, physical therapists, and patients is key to designing safe and effective exercise and rehabilitation programs that align with treatment objectives and individual needs. By incorporating exercise and rehabilitation into thymic tumor care, patients can enhance their overall health and resilience throughout their cancer journey.

8.4 Mind-Body Approaches: Stress Reduction and Psychological Support for Thymic Tumor Patients

Coping with a thymic tumor diagnosis can be emotionally challenging, and addressing the psychological and emotional well-being of patients is an essential aspect of comprehensive care. Mind-body approaches, including stress reduction techniques and psychological support, play a crucial role in helping thymic tumor patients manage the emotional impact of their diagnosis, improve their quality of life, and enhance their overall well-being. In this section, we will explore the significance of mind-body approaches in thymic tumor care and discuss various strategies to promote emotional and psychological health.

1. Understanding the Emotional Impact:

Receiving a thymic tumor diagnosis can evoke a range of emotions, including fear, anxiety, sadness, anger, and uncertainty. The emotional impact extends beyond the patient to their families and caregivers. Acknowledging and addressing these emotions is essential to providing holistic care.

a. Anxiety and Fear: The uncertainty of a cancer diagnosis, treatment outcomes, and potential side effects can lead to heightened anxiety and fear.

b. Depression: Coping with a serious illness can contribute to depression, which may manifest as persistent sadness, loss of interest in activities, and changes in sleep and appetite.

c. Stress: The demands of cancer treatment, medical appointments, and lifestyle adjustments can lead to chronic stress, which can affect physical health and overall well-being.

d. Impact on Relationships: A thymic tumor diagnosis can strain relationships with loved ones and caregivers, leading to additional emotional challenges.

e. Coping with Trauma: Some patients may experience trauma related to their cancer journey, especially if they have undergone major surgeries or faced life-threatening complications.

2. Benefits of Mind-Body Approaches:

Mind-body approaches encompass a range of techniques and practices that focus on the connection between the mind, emotions, and the body. These approaches offer several potential benefits for thymic tumor patients:

a. Stress Reduction: Mind-body techniques can reduce stress and promote relaxation, leading to improved overall well-being.

b. Emotional Regulation: These approaches can help patients better cope with difficult emotions, manage anxiety, and reduce symptoms of depression.

c. Pain Management: Mind-body techniques can complement pain management strategies, reducing the need for pain medication.

d. Enhanced Quality of Life: By improving emotional well-being, mind-body approaches contribute to an improved quality of life and overall satisfaction.

e. Support for Coping Strategies: Patients can learn effective coping strategies and resilience-building techniques to navigate the challenges of their cancer journey.

3. Mind-Body Approaches for Thymic Tumor Patients:

A variety of mind-body approaches can be beneficial for thymic tumor patients, including:

a. Mindfulness Meditation: Mindfulness meditation involves paying focused attention to the present moment, reducing anxiety and promoting emotional regulation.

b. Relaxation Techniques: Deep breathing exercises, progressive muscle relaxation, and guided imagery can induce relaxation and reduce stress.

c. Yoga: Yoga combines physical postures, breathing exercises, and meditation to enhance physical and emotional well-being.

d. Tai Chi: Tai chi is a gentle, slow-moving exercise that can improve balance, flexibility, and emotional resilience.

e. Art Therapy: Engaging in creative activities such as painting, drawing, or sculpture provides an outlet for self-expression and emotional processing.

f. Music Therapy: Music therapy involves using music to reduce stress, manage emotions, and improve mood.

g. Supportive Counseling: Counseling, including individual therapy, group therapy, and family counseling, can provide a safe space for patients to discuss their feelings and challenges.

h. Support Groups: Support groups connect patients with others facing similar experiences, providing a sense of community and shared understanding.

i. Cognitive-Behavioral Therapy (CBT): CBT is a structured therapeutic approach that helps patients identify and modify negative thought patterns and behaviors.

4. Implementing Mind-Body Approaches:

Integrating mind-body approaches into the care of thymic tumor patients requires a comprehensive and patient-centered approach:

a. Patient Assessment: Healthcare providers should assess the emotional and psychological needs of patients and provide appropriate referrals to mind-body services.

b. Individualized Plans: Treatment plans should be tailored to the unique needs and preferences of each patient, taking into account their emotional state and coping strategies.

c. Collaborative Care: A multidisciplinary team, including oncologists, psychologists, social workers, and mind-body practitioners, can work together to provide holistic care.

d. Education: Patients and their families should receive education on available mind-body techniques and their potential benefits.

e. Accessibility: Efforts should be made to ensure that mind-body services are accessible to all patients, regardless of their location or financial resources.

5. Psychological Support and Counseling:

Psychological support is a fundamental component of mind-body approaches for thymic tumor patients:

a. Individual Counseling: Individual counseling provides a safe and confidential space for patients to explore their emotions, develop coping strategies, and address specific psychological challenges.

b. Group Therapy: Group therapy sessions allow patients to connect with others who share similar experiences, fostering a sense of community and mutual support.

c. Family Counseling: Thymic tumor diagnoses can impact the entire family. Family counseling helps address family dynamics and provides tools for effective communication and support.

d. Coping Skills Training: Psychologists can teach patients coping skills and stress management techniques to navigate the emotional challenges of cancer.

e. Crisis Intervention: In times of acute distress or crisis, immediate psychological support and crisis intervention should be available.

6. Survivorship and Long-Term Well-Being:

The emotional impact of cancer does not end with treatment. Mind-body approaches continue to be valuable during survivorship:

a. Survivorship Care Plans: Survivorship care plans should include recommendations for ongoing psychological support and mind-body practices to address late effects and emotional well-being.

b. Monitoring Emotional Health: Regular assessments of emotional health and quality of life can help detect and address psychological concerns in the long term.

c. Coping with Late Effects: Patients should receive support and strategies for coping with late effects of treatment, which may impact emotional well-being.

d. Support for Fertility and Hormonal Health: Adolescent and young adult survivors may require counseling on fertility preservation and addressing hormonal health.

e. Educational and Vocational Support: Adolescents and young adults should receive support for pursuing their educational and vocational goals, considering their emotional well-being.

7. Conclusion:

Mind-body approaches, including stress reduction techniques and psychological support, are integral components of thymic tumor care that address the emotional and psychological well-being of patients. These approaches offer a range of potential benefits, including stress reduction, emotional regulation, pain management, and improved quality of life. Implementing mind-body approaches requires a patient-centered and collaborative approach, with healthcare providers, psychologists, and mind-body practitioners working together to meet the unique emotional needs of each patient. By incorporating these strategies into thymic tumor care, patients can better manage the emotional challenges of their cancer journey and enhance their overall well-being and resilience.

8.5 Complementary Therapies and Their Role in Thymic Tumor Care

Complementary therapies, often referred to as integrative or alternative therapies, have gained recognition as valuable adjuncts to conventional medical treatments in cancer care. These therapies encompass a wide range of practices and approaches that can play a significant role in enhancing the overall well-being of thymic tumor patients. In this section, we will explore the role of complementary therapies in thymic tumor care, their potential benefits, and considerations for their safe and effective integration into treatment plans.

1. Understanding Complementary Therapies:

Complementary therapies are approaches that are used alongside conventional medical treatments to support the physical, emotional, and psychological well-being of patients. They are typically considered complementary when used in conjunction with standard medical care and alternative when used as a substitute for conventional treatments, which is generally discouraged in cancer care.

2. Potential Benefits of Complementary Therapies:

Complementary therapies offer several potential benefits for thymic tumor patients:

a. Symptom Management: Many complementary therapies can help manage treatment-related symptoms such as pain, nausea, fatigue, and anxiety.

b. Improved Quality of Life: These therapies may enhance the overall quality of life by reducing distress, improving mood, and promoting a sense of well-being.

c. Stress Reduction: Practices like meditation, yoga, and relaxation techniques can reduce stress, which is a common concern among cancer patients.

d. Enhanced Immune Function: Some complementary therapies, such as acupuncture and certain dietary supplements, are believed to support immune function.

e. Pain Relief: Techniques like acupuncture, massage therapy, and chiropractic care may help alleviate pain and discomfort.

f. Support for Emotional Health: Complementary therapies can provide emotional support and promote emotional resilience during the cancer journey.

3. Types of Complementary Therapies:

Complementary therapies encompass a diverse array of practices and interventions, including but not limited to:

a. Mind-Body Practices:

1. **Meditation:** Mindfulness meditation, guided imagery, and other meditation techniques can reduce stress and promote emotional well-being.
2. **Yoga:** Yoga combines physical postures, breathing

exercises, and meditation to enhance physical and emotional health.
3. **Tai Chi:** Tai chi is a gentle, slow-moving exercise that improves balance, flexibility, and emotional resilience.

b. **Body-Based Practices:**

1. **Massage Therapy:** Massage can alleviate muscle tension, reduce pain, and promote relaxation.
2. **Chiropractic Care:** Chiropractic adjustments may help manage musculoskeletal discomfort and improve overall well-being.
3. **Acupuncture:** Acupuncture involves the insertion of thin needles into specific points on the body to relieve pain and reduce symptoms.

c. **Energy-Based Therapies:**

1. **Reiki:** Reiki is a form of energy healing that aims to balance the body's energy and promote relaxation.
2. **Therapeutic Touch:** Therapeutic touch involves the practitioner's hands hovering over the patient's body to channel healing energy.

d. **Dietary and Nutritional Interventions:**

1. **Dietary Supplements:** Some patients may explore the use of dietary supplements, such as vitamins, minerals, and herbs, to support their health.
2. **Nutritional Counseling:** Nutritionists can provide guidance on dietary choices to optimize health during treatment and recovery.

e. **Herbal Medicine:**

1. **Traditional Herbal Remedies:** Some patients may use traditional herbal remedies as complementary

therapies. It is crucial for healthcare providers to be aware of these practices to ensure safety and monitor potential interactions with conventional treatments.

f. Aromatherapy:

1. **Essential Oils:** Aromatherapy involves the use of essential oils, often in combination with massage or diffusion, to promote relaxation and emotional well-being.

g. Art and Music Therapy:

1. **Art Therapy:** Creative expression through art can provide an outlet for emotional processing and stress reduction.
2. **Music Therapy:** Music therapy uses music to reduce stress, improve mood, and enhance emotional well-being.

4. Integrating Complementary Therapies:

Integrating complementary therapies into thymic tumor care requires a patient-centered and collaborative approach:

a. Patient Education: Patients should be informed about available complementary therapies, their potential benefits, and their role in the overall treatment plan.

b. Individualized Treatment Plans: Complementary therapies should be tailored to the unique needs, preferences, and medical history of each patient.

c. Collaboration: A multidisciplinary team, including oncologists, nurses, and complementary therapy practitioners, should collaborate to ensure safe and effective integration.

d. Communication: Open communication between

patients, healthcare providers, and complementary therapy practitioners is essential to coordinate care and monitor progress.

e. **Safety Precautions:** Complementary therapies should be used with awareness of potential risks and contraindications, especially in patients undergoing specific cancer treatments.

f. **Research and Evidence-Based Practices:** Whenever possible, complementary therapies should be selected based on scientific evidence of their effectiveness and safety.

5. Symptom Management and Support:

Complementary therapies can be particularly valuable for managing specific symptoms and side effects experienced by thymic tumor patients:

a. **Pain Management:** Acupuncture, massage therapy, and chiropractic care may help alleviate cancer-related pain.

b. **Nausea and Vomiting:** Acupuncture, aromatherapy, and dietary modifications may reduce treatment-induced nausea and vomiting.

c. **Fatigue:** Mind-body practices like meditation and yoga can improve energy levels and reduce cancer-related fatigue.

d. **Anxiety and Depression:** Mindfulness meditation, art therapy, and music therapy can support emotional well-being and help manage anxiety and depression.

6. Survivorship and Long-Term Well-Being:

Complementary therapies can continue to play a role in thymic tumor care during the survivorship phase:

a. **Survivorship Care Plans:** Survivorship care plans may include recommendations for ongoing complementary therapies to address late effects, emotional well-being, and long-term health.

b. Monitoring and Assessments: Regular assessments of symptom management and emotional health can help detect and address ongoing concerns.

c. Coping with Late Effects: Complementary therapies can be used to manage late effects of treatment, such as pain, fatigue, and emotional distress.

d. Support for Long-Term Well-Being: Patients should be encouraged to incorporate complementary therapies into their long-term health and well-being strategies.

7. Conclusion:

Complementary therapies have a valuable role to play in thymic tumor care by addressing symptoms, enhancing quality of life, and providing emotional and psychological support to patients. These therapies should be integrated into the treatment plan with careful consideration of individual patient needs, preferences, and safety. A collaborative approach involving healthcare providers, complementary therapy practitioners, and patients is essential to ensure that complementary therapies align with treatment objectives and contribute to the holistic care of thymic tumor patients. By incorporating these approaches into thymic tumor care, patients can access a broader range of tools and resources to support their well-being throughout their cancer journey.

8.6 Holistic Approaches to Survivorship Care for Thymic Tumor Patients

Survivorship care for thymic tumor patients extends beyond medical treatment and addresses their physical, emotional, psychological, and social well-being. Holistic approaches to survivorship care emphasize the integration of various aspects of health, aiming to optimize the overall quality of life and long-term well-being of patients. In this section, we will explore holistic survivorship care for thymic tumor patients, covering physical health, emotional support, lifestyle considerations, and the importance of ongoing monitoring and care.

1. The Concept of Holistic Survivorship Care:

Holistic survivorship care recognizes that the journey of cancer survivors involves multifaceted challenges and opportunities for growth. This approach focuses on addressing the physical, emotional, psychological, and social aspects of survivorship.

2. Physical Health and Monitoring:

a. **Regular Follow-Up Appointments:** Thymic tumor survivors should have regular follow-up appointments with their oncologists or specialists to monitor their health and detect any potential recurrence or late effects of treatment.

b. **Imaging and Testing:** Periodic imaging scans and laboratory tests may be recommended to monitor for any signs of cancer recurrence or long-term treatment-related complications.

c. **Cardiovascular Health:** Thymic tumors and certain treatments can affect cardiovascular health. Holistic survivorship care includes monitoring for heart-related issues and providing interventions as needed.

d. **Lung Function:** As the thymus is located near the lungs, monitoring lung function is crucial, especially for patients who have undergone surgery or radiation therapy.

3. Emotional and Psychological Support:

a. **Psychological Assessment:** Regular psychological assessments can identify any emotional distress, anxiety, depression, or post-traumatic stress that survivors may experience.

b. **Counseling and Therapy:** Survivorship care includes access to counseling and therapy services to help patients cope with emotional challenges and develop effective strategies for managing stress and anxiety.

c. **Support Groups:** Thymic tumor survivors benefit from participation in support groups, where they can connect with others who share similar experiences and find peer support.

d. **Mind-Body Practices:** Mindfulness meditation, yoga, and other mind-body practices can promote emotional well-being, reduce stress, and support psychological resilience.

4. Lifestyle Considerations:

a. **Healthy Diet:** Encouraging survivors to maintain a balanced and nutritious diet can promote overall health, energy levels, and the management of late effects.

b. **Physical Activity:** Physical activity tailored to individual capabilities helps survivors maintain or improve physical function, reduce fatigue, and support cardiovascular health.

c. **Smoking Cessation:** Smoking cessation programs are essential, especially for those who were smokers before their diagnosis, to reduce the risk of further health complications.

d. **Alcohol Moderation:** Guidance on alcohol moderation or cessation, depending on individual health and lifestyle factors, is part of holistic survivorship care.

e. **Sleep Hygiene:** Addressing sleep disturbances and promoting good sleep hygiene can enhance physical and emotional well-being.

f. **Stress Reduction:** Stress management techniques, such as relaxation exercises, can help survivors cope with stress and reduce the risk of stress-related health issues.

5. Rehabilitation and Physical Function:

a. **Physical Rehabilitation:** Physical rehabilitation programs help survivors regain physical function, address muscle weakness, and manage mobility challenges, especially after surgery.

b. **Occupational Therapy:** Occupational therapy focuses on helping survivors regain independence in daily activities and return to work or other meaningful roles.

6. Addressing Late Effects:

a. **Late Effects Management:** Survivors may experience late effects of treatment, such as cardiac issues, lung problems, or hormonal imbalances. Holistic survivorship care includes the management of these late effects to optimize overall health.

b. **Fertility and Hormonal Health:** Young adult survivors may require specialized care for fertility preservation and management of hormonal health, particularly if treatment affected their reproductive system.

c. **Pain Management:** Holistic care addresses pain management strategies, including physical therapy, medications, and complementary therapies, to improve comfort and function.

7. Survivorship Care Plans:

a. **Individualized Plans:** Each thymic tumor survivor should have an individualized survivorship care plan that considers their unique medical history, treatment journey, and specific needs.

b. **Care Coordination:** Survivorship care plans involve care coordination among oncologists, primary care providers, specialists, and other healthcare professionals.

c. **Psychosocial Care:** The plan includes psychosocial care, encompassing emotional support, counseling, and access to mental health services.

d. **Lifestyle Recommendations:** Lifestyle recommendations are part of the plan, emphasizing the importance of a healthy diet, regular exercise, and smoking cessation.

e. **Monitoring and Surveillance:** The plan outlines a schedule for ongoing monitoring and surveillance to detect any potential issues early.

8. Long-Term Well-Being:

a. **Health Promotion:** Holistic survivorship care promotes long-term health and well-being by providing guidance on maintaining a healthy lifestyle and reducing the risk of chronic health conditions.

b. **Cancer Screening:** Survivors may be at an increased risk of other cancers. Holistic care includes age-appropriate cancer screening recommendations.

c. **Emotional Resilience:** Programs and interventions that foster emotional resilience and coping skills are integral to long-term well-being.

d. **Social Support:** Social support networks, including family, friends, and support groups, play a significant role in the long-term emotional and psychological health of survivors.

9. Survivorship Care Navigation:

a. **Navigation Services:** Survivorship care navigation services help survivors navigate the healthcare system, access resources, and understand their survivorship care plan.

b. **Communication:** Navigators facilitate communication between survivors and their healthcare providers, ensuring that the survivor's needs are understood and addressed.

c. **Education:** Providing survivors with information about survivorship care, late effects, and self-care practices is a core component of navigation services.

10. Palliative and End-of-Life Care:

a. **Palliative Care:** For those with advanced-stage thymic tumors or other life-limiting conditions, palliative care ensures that symptom management, comfort, and quality of life remain the focus of care.

b. **End-of-Life Care:** Holistic care also includes end-of-life care planning, which involves discussions about preferences for care, advanced directives, and support for both patients and their families.

11. Survivorship Research:

a. **Research Opportunities:** Holistic survivorship care includes research initiatives aimed at improving survivorship outcomes, understanding late effects, and enhancing the long-term well-being of thymic tumor survivors.

12. Conclusion:

Holistic approaches to survivorship care for thymic tumor patients recognize the complexity of the survivorship journey and address the physical, emotional, psychological, and social aspects of survivorship. By providing comprehensive care that extends beyond the medical aspects of treatment, healthcare providers can empower survivors to optimize their overall quality of life, emotional well-being, and long-term health. Survivorship care plans, lifestyle considerations, late effects management, and ongoing monitoring are all essential components of this holistic approach. Through collaboration between healthcare professionals, support networks, and survivors themselves, holistic survivorship care can help individuals thrive in their post-cancer journey, finding meaning, purpose, and resilience in the face of adversity.

CHAPTER 9: ADVANCES IN IMAGING AND DIAGNOSTICS

9.1 Cutting-Edge Imaging Modalities in Thymic Tumor Diagnosis and Monitoring

In the field of thymic tumors, advanced imaging modalities have revolutionized the diagnosis, staging, and monitoring of patients. These cutting-edge technologies provide clinicians with detailed insights into tumor characteristics, response to treatment, and potential complications. In this section, we will explore the latest advancements in imaging modalities and their critical role in managing thymic tumors.

1. Imaging in Thymic Tumors:

Imaging plays a pivotal role in the management of thymic tumors, serving multiple purposes:

a. **Diagnosis:** Imaging helps identify the presence of a thymic tumor, its location, size, and potential involvement of adjacent structures.

b. **Staging:** Accurate staging is crucial for treatment planning. Imaging determines the extent of tumor spread, lymph node involvement, and distant metastasis.

c. **Treatment Planning:** Imaging guides surgical planning, radiation therapy, and chemotherapy strategies.

d. **Monitoring:** After treatment initiation, imaging tracks tumor response, detects recurrence, and evaluates treatment-related complications.

2. Conventional Imaging Techniques:

a. **Chest X-rays:** Traditional chest X-rays provide an initial overview of the thymus and any potential abnormalities. However, they lack the detail required for precise diagnosis and staging.

b. **Computed Tomography (CT):** CT scans offer higher-resolution images, aiding in the characterization and staging of thymic tumors. Advances in CT technology, such as multi-detector CT, have improved image quality and reduced scan times.

c. **Magnetic Resonance Imaging (MRI):** MRI is valuable for assessing thymic tumors, especially in cases where radiation exposure is a concern (e.g., young patients). It provides excellent soft tissue contrast but may require longer scan times.

d. **Positron Emission Tomography (PET):** PET scans, often combined with CT (PET/CT), help detect metabolic activity in thymic tumors and identify metastatic lesions elsewhere in the body. Fluorodeoxyglucose (FDG) is the most commonly used radiotracer.

3. Cutting-Edge Imaging Modalities:

Recent advancements in imaging technologies have expanded the capabilities of thymic tumor diagnosis and monitoring. These cutting-edge modalities offer greater accuracy, earlier detection, and improved treatment planning.

a. Magnetic Resonance Imaging with Diffusion-Weighted Imaging (DWI-MRI):

- **Principle:** DWI-MRI measures the diffusion of water molecules within tissues. Tumor tissues typically have restricted water diffusion compared to healthy tissues.
- **Advantages:** It provides detailed information about tumor cellularity and can help differentiate thymic tumors from other mediastinal masses. DWI-MRI is particularly useful for monitoring treatment response.

b. Dynamic Contrast-Enhanced MRI (DCE-MRI):

- **Principle:** DCE-MRI tracks the flow of a contrast agent (usually gadolinium-based) through blood vessels and tissues over time. This information helps assess tumor vascularity and perfusion.
- **Advantages:** DCE-MRI can distinguish between benign and malignant thymic tumors and provide insights into angiogenesis, which is critical for tumor growth and spread.

c. Chest Magnetic Resonance Imaging with Integrated Parallel Imaging Techniques (e.g., 3T MRI):

- **Principle:** High-field MRI (e.g., 3 Tesla) provides enhanced image resolution and signal-to-noise ratio, improving the visualization of small lesions and anatomical details.
- **Advantages:** 3T MRI can be particularly beneficial for detecting small thymic tumors, characterizing tumor boundaries, and assessing potential invasion into neighboring structures.

d. Perfusion Imaging Techniques:

- **Principle:** Perfusion imaging, including arterial spin labeling (ASL) and dynamic susceptibility contrast (DSC) MRI, measures blood flow within tissues, aiding in the evaluation of tumor vascularity.
- **Advantages:** These techniques provide valuable information about tumor blood supply and may assist in differentiating thymic tumors from other mediastinal masses.

e. 3D-Printed Models for Surgical Planning:

- **Principle:** 3D printing technology generates anatomical models based on patient-specific imaging data. Surgeons can use these models to plan complex thymic tumor resections.
- **Advantages:** 3D-printed models enhance surgical precision by allowing surgeons to practice procedures on patient-specific anatomical replicas before the actual operation.

f. Radiomics and Machine Learning:

- **Principle:** Radiomics involves the extraction of quantitative data from medical images, such as texture features, which can be analyzed using machine learning algorithms to predict tumor characteristics, treatment response, and patient outcomes.
- **Advantages:** Radiomics and machine learning hold promise in improving diagnostic accuracy, treatment planning, and prognostication for thymic tumors.

g. Novel PET Tracers (e.g., Ga-68 DOTATATE):

- **Principle:** Ga-68 DOTATATE PET scans target somatostatin receptor expression, which can be elevated in neuroendocrine thymic tumors.
- **Advantages:** Ga-68 DOTATATE PET offers superior

sensitivity in detecting thymic neuroendocrine tumors compared to FDG-PET and can guide treatment decisions.

4. Personalized Imaging and Treatment Planning:

These cutting-edge imaging modalities enable more personalized approaches to thymic tumor management:

a. **Radiogenomics:** The integration of radiomic features with genomic data can help identify imaging-genomic associations, offering insights into tumor biology and treatment response prediction.

b. **Theranostics:** Combining diagnostic imaging with targeted therapy is a promising approach. For example, certain PET tracers can identify targets for radionuclide therapy in thymic tumors.

c. **Precision Radiation Therapy:** Advanced imaging techniques assist in precise radiation therapy planning, minimizing radiation exposure to adjacent healthy tissues.

5. Challenges and Considerations:

a. **Cost and Accessibility:** Some cutting-edge imaging modalities may be costly or less accessible in certain healthcare settings, posing challenges for widespread adoption.

b. **Radiation Exposure:** While imaging is crucial, clinicians must consider the cumulative radiation exposure, particularly in young patients who may require long-term monitoring.

c. **Interdisciplinary Collaboration:** Interpretation of advanced imaging data often necessitates collaboration between radiologists, oncologists, and other specialists to optimize patient care.

6. Future Directions:

Continued research and development in imaging technologies for thymic tumors hold promise for:

a. **Early Detection:** Improved imaging may enable earlier detection of thymic tumors, potentially leading to better outcomes.

b. **Personalized Treatment:** Advanced imaging can inform personalized treatment strategies, minimizing side effects and optimizing therapeutic efficacy.

c. **Outcome Prediction:** Further integration of radiomics, genomics, and clinical data may enhance the prediction of treatment response and long-term outcomes.

7. Conclusion:

Cutting-edge imaging modalities have transformed the diagnosis, staging, and monitoring of thymic tumors, providing clinicians with valuable insights into tumor characteristics and treatment responses. From advanced MRI techniques to novel PET tracers and 3D-printed surgical models, these innovations offer opportunities for early detection, personalized treatment planning, and improved patient outcomes. As technology continues to advance, the field of thymic tumor imaging holds great promise for enhancing the care and quality of life of patients facing these complex malignancies.

9.2 Molecular Imaging and PET/CT in Thymic Tumors: Advancements and Clinical Applications

Molecular imaging, particularly through the use of Positron Emission Tomography combined with Computed Tomography (PET/CT), has emerged as a powerful tool in the management of thymic tumors. This advanced imaging modality provides valuable molecular and functional information, enabling clinicians to enhance diagnosis, staging, treatment planning, and monitoring. In this section, we will explore the role of molecular imaging, with a focus on PET/CT, in thymic tumors, including its principles, clinical applications, and recent advancements.

1. Molecular Imaging and PET/CT:

Molecular imaging is a branch of medical imaging that visualizes molecular and cellular processes within the body. It goes beyond traditional anatomical imaging (such as CT and MRI) by providing insights into the biological activity of tissues. PET/CT combines Positron Emission Tomography (PET) and Computed Tomography (CT) into a single imaging session, allowing the simultaneous assessment of both anatomical and molecular information. In thymic tumors, molecular imaging plays a pivotal role in improving diagnosis, staging, and treatment monitoring.

2. Principles of PET/CT Imaging:

- **PET:** PET involves the administration of a radiopharmaceutical, typically Fluorine-18 Fluorodeoxyglucose (18F-FDG), which is a glucose analog labeled with a radioactive isotope. Cancer cells are often more metabolically active and take up more glucose than normal cells. When a patient receives the radiopharmaceutical, the PET scanner detects gamma-ray emissions produced by the radiotracer's decay. Areas with high radiotracer uptake indicate increased metabolic activity, which is typical of cancerous tissue.
- **CT:** CT provides detailed anatomical images using X-rays. By combining PET and CT, PET/CT allows for precise localization of the areas of increased metabolic activity within the context of the patient's anatomy.

3. Clinical Applications of PET/CT in Thymic Tumors:

PET/CT has a wide range of clinical applications in thymic tumors:

a. **Diagnosis:** PET/CT aids in differentiating thymic tumors from other mediastinal masses. It can identify malignant thymic tumors based on their increased 18F-FDG uptake.

b. **Staging:** Accurate staging is crucial for treatment planning. PET/CT helps determine the extent of tumor spread, involvement of adjacent structures, and the presence of distant metastases.

c. **Treatment Planning:** PET/CT plays a vital role in surgical planning, radiation therapy, and chemotherapy strategies by providing information on tumor location, size, and metabolic activity.

d. **Response Assessment:** After treatment initiation, PET/CT assesses tumor response to therapy. A decrease in metabolic activity often indicates a positive response, while persistent or increased activity may suggest treatment resistance.

e. **Recurrence Detection:** PET/CT is sensitive to small lesions and is valuable for detecting tumor recurrence, even at an early stage.

f. **Monitoring Complications:** PET/CT can identify and monitor treatment-related complications, such as radiation-induced lung injury or cardiac toxicity.

4. Advancements in PET/CT for Thymic Tumors:

Recent advancements in PET/CT technology and techniques have further improved its utility in thymic tumors:

a. **Quantitative PET Imaging:** Quantitative analysis of PET images, including standardized uptake values (SUVs) and metabolic tumor volume (MTV), provides more accurate measurements of tumor activity and facilitates treatment response assessment.

b. **Dual-Time-Point Imaging:** Dual-time-point PET/CT, which involves imaging at two different time intervals after radiotracer injection, can distinguish between malignant and benign thymic lesions based on their temporal changes in 18F-FDG uptake.

c. **Advanced PET Tracers:** Beyond 18F-FDG, new PET tracers are being explored for thymic tumors. For example, Ga-68 DOTATATE targets somatostatin receptors and is particularly useful in thymic neuroendocrine tumors.

d. **Artificial Intelligence (AI):** AI-driven algorithms are being developed to improve the accuracy of lesion detection and quantitative analysis in PET/CT images, enhancing diagnostic and prognostic capabilities.

e. **Personalized Treatment Planning:** PET/CT data are increasingly integrated with treatment planning systems, allowing for more precise radiation therapy and targeted therapies.

5. Challenges and Considerations:

Despite its numerous advantages, PET/CT in thymic tumors presents certain challenges:

a. **Radiation Exposure:** PET/CT involves exposure to ionizing radiation, which must be carefully considered, especially in pediatric or young adult patients who may require long-term monitoring.

b. **False Positives:** Inflammation, infection, or other benign conditions can sometimes lead to false-positive PET/

CT findings, necessitating further evaluation and potential biopsy.

c. **Interpretation:** Accurate interpretation of PET/CT images requires expertise in both oncology and nuclear medicine. Multidisciplinary collaboration among radiologists, oncologists, and nuclear medicine specialists is essential.

d. **Cost:** PET/CT can be relatively expensive compared to other imaging modalities, and its availability may be limited in some healthcare settings.

6. Future Directions:

The future of molecular imaging and PET/CT in thymic tumors holds promising developments:

a. **Radiomics and AI:** The integration of radiomics and AI in PET/CT analysis is expected to improve the predictive power of imaging for treatment response and outcomes.

b. **Novel Radiotracers:** The development of novel PET tracers specific to thymic tumor subtypes may further enhance diagnostic accuracy and treatment selection.

c. **Reduced Radiation Exposure:** Ongoing research aims to reduce radiation exposure in PET/CT, making it safer for patients, especially in long-term monitoring scenarios.

7. Conclusion:

Molecular imaging, particularly through PET/CT, has transformed the management of thymic tumors. By providing both anatomical and molecular information, PET/CT enhances diagnosis, staging, treatment planning, and monitoring. Recent advancements in quantitative analysis, dual-time-point imaging, novel PET tracers, AI, and personalized treatment planning have further improved its clinical utility. While challenges such as radiation exposure and false positives exist, the future of PET/CT in thymic tumors holds exciting opportunities for improved patient care and outcomes. This advanced imaging modality continues to play a crucial role in the multidisciplinary approach to thymic tumor management, ultimately benefiting patients by guiding treatment decisions and optimizing therapeutic strategies.

9.3 Liquid Biopsies and Circulating Tumor Markers in Thymic Tumors: A Paradigm Shift in Diagnosis and Monitoring

Liquid biopsies have emerged as a revolutionary approach in the field of oncology, offering a minimally invasive means to detect and monitor cancer. Thymic tumors, a relatively rare group of malignancies, are no exception to the transformative potential of liquid biopsies. In this section, we will explore the concept of liquid biopsies, the significance of circulating tumor markers, their clinical applications in thymic tumors, and recent advancements in this promising field.

1. Liquid Biopsies:

Liquid biopsies represent a paradigm shift in cancer diagnosis and monitoring. Unlike traditional tissue biopsies, which involve the surgical removal of tissue samples, liquid biopsies analyze various biomarkers present in bodily fluids such as blood (circulating tumor DNA, ctDNA), plasma, serum, urine, and cerebrospinal fluid. Liquid biopsies offer several advantages:

- **Minimally Invasive:** Liquid biopsies can be obtained through a simple blood draw, reducing the need for invasive procedures.
- **Real-time Monitoring:** They enable real-time monitoring of tumor dynamics, treatment response, and the emergence of resistance.

- **Early Detection:** Liquid biopsies have the potential to detect cancer at earlier stages, improving treatment outcomes.
- **Tumor Heterogeneity:** Liquid biopsies can capture the genetic diversity of tumors, which may be missed in a single tissue biopsy.
- **Patient Convenience:** They are less burdensome for patients, allowing for more frequent testing.

2. Circulating Tumor Markers in Thymic Tumors:

Circulating tumor markers are substances released by cancer cells into the bloodstream. In thymic tumors, several types of circulating tumor markers have been studied, including:

- **Circulating Tumor DNA (ctDNA):** ctDNA is fragments of tumor DNA that are shed into the bloodstream as cancer cells die. It contains genetic mutations specific to the tumor, providing valuable information about tumor genetics and evolution.
- **Circulating Tumor Cells (CTCs):** CTCs are intact cancer cells that have detached from the primary tumor and entered the bloodstream. They can be isolated and analyzed to understand tumor biology and metastatic potential.
- **Cancer-associated Proteins:** Proteins produced by thymic tumors, such as CEA (Carcinoembryonic Antigen) and NSE (Neuron-Specific Enolase), can be detected in the blood and serve as biomarkers.

3. Clinical Applications of Liquid Biopsies in Thymic Tumors:

Liquid biopsies have several clinical applications in thymic tumors:

a. Diagnosis: Liquid biopsies can aid in the diagnosis of thymic tumors by detecting specific genetic mutations or tumor-specific biomarkers in the bloodstream. This is especially valuable when obtaining tissue biopsies is challenging or when confirming the diagnosis of thymic carcinomas.

b. Staging: Circulating tumor markers can provide insights into the extent of disease and potential for metastasis. Elevated levels of certain markers may indicate a more advanced stage of thymic tumors.

c. Treatment Selection: Liquid biopsies can identify actionable mutations or genetic alterations that guide treatment decisions. For example, the presence of specific mutations may make a patient eligible for targeted therapies.

d. Treatment Response Monitoring: Serial liquid biopsies allow for real-time monitoring of treatment response. Changes in ctDNA levels or genetic mutations can indicate whether a treatment is effective or if resistance is developing.

e. Early Detection of Recurrence: Liquid biopsies are sensitive to minimal residual disease (MRD) and can detect tumor recurrence earlier than traditional imaging methods.

f. Tumor Heterogeneity: Liquid biopsies capture the genetic diversity of thymic tumors, helping clinicians understand the full spectrum of tumor mutations and adapt treatment accordingly.

4. Recent Advancements in Liquid Biopsies for Thymic Tumors:

Recent advancements in liquid biopsies have expanded their utility in thymic tumors:

a. Next-Generation Sequencing (NGS): NGS technologies have enhanced the ability to detect a wide range of genetic alterations in ctDNA, providing a comprehensive genetic profile of thymic tumors.

b. Digital PCR: Digital PCR techniques enable highly sensitive and quantitative detection of specific mutations or biomarkers in ctDNA, allowing for precise treatment monitoring.

c. Multi-omic Analysis: Integrating data from different omics platforms, including genomics, transcriptomics, and proteomics, provides a more comprehensive understanding of tumor biology.

d. Machine Learning: Machine learning algorithms can analyze complex liquid biopsy data to identify patterns, predict treatment responses, and stratify patients based on risk.

e. Circulating RNA: Beyond ctDNA, circulating RNA molecules, such as microRNAs and long non-coding RNAs, are emerging as valuable biomarkers in thymic tumors.

f. Exosome Analysis: Exosomes, small vesicles secreted by tumor cells, carry genetic material and proteins that can be analyzed to gain insights into tumor communication and progression.

5. Challenges and Considerations:

Despite their potential, liquid biopsies in thymic tumors come with certain challenges:

a. Sensitivity: The sensitivity of liquid biopsies can vary among patients and tumor types. Some tumors may shed less ctDNA or CTCs into the bloodstream, making detection more challenging.

b. Specificity: Ensuring that detected genetic alterations are truly tumor-specific and not related to other conditions or benign lesions is crucial.

c. Standardization: Standardizing liquid biopsy procedures, including sample collection, processing, and analysis, is essential to ensure reliability and reproducibility.

d. Clinical Validation: Many liquid biopsy tests are still in the experimental or research phase and require rigorous clinical validation before widespread clinical use.

e. Cost and Accessibility: Liquid biopsy testing, particularly comprehensive NGS, can be costly, and accessibility may be limited in some healthcare settings.

6. Future Directions:

The future of liquid biopsies in thymic tumors holds exciting possibilities:

a. Early Detection and Prevention: Liquid biopsies may enable the early detection of thymic tumors in high-risk individuals, allowing for timely intervention and potentially preventing disease progression.

b. Personalized Treatment: Advanced liquid biopsy techniques will continue to guide the selection of targeted therapies and inform treatment decisions tailored to individual patients.

c. Biomarker Discovery: Ongoing research will uncover new circulating tumor markers and biomarkers that offer insights into thymic tumor biology and therapeutic vulnerabilities.

d. Integration with Imaging: Combining liquid biopsy data with advanced imaging modalities, such as PET/CT, will provide a more comprehensive view of tumor characteristics and dynamics.

7. Conclusion:

Liquid biopsies and circulating tumor markers have revolutionized the diagnosis and management of thymic tumors. These minimally invasive techniques offer invaluable insights into tumor genetics, treatment response, and early detection of recurrence. Recent advancements in technology, including NGS, digital PCR, multi-omic analysis, and machine learning, have expanded the capabilities of liquid biopsies in thymic tumors. While challenges remain, ongoing research and clinical validation efforts promise to further enhance the role of liquid biopsies in improving patient outcomes and quality of life in thymic tumor care.

9.4 Radiomics and Artificial Intelligence in Thymic Tumors: Revolutionizing Diagnosis and Treatment

Radiomics and Artificial Intelligence (AI) have emerged as transformative technologies in the field of oncology, offering a data-driven approach to medical imaging analysis. In the context of thymic tumors, radiomics and AI are poised to revolutionize diagnosis, prognosis, treatment planning, and monitoring. This section explores the principles, clinical applications, recent advancements, challenges, and the promising future of radiomics and AI in thymic tumors.

1. Radiomics and Artificial Intelligence:

- **Radiomics:** Radiomics is a discipline that extracts a vast amount of quantitative data from medical images, such as CT scans or MRI images. These data include texture features, shape characteristics, and intensity patterns within a tumor and its surrounding tissues. Radiomics aims to uncover hidden information in medical images that may not be visible to the human eye.
- **Artificial Intelligence:** AI involves the use of computer

algorithms and machine learning techniques to process and analyze complex medical data, including radiomics features. AI can identify patterns, make predictions, and assist in clinical decision-making based on the information it learns from large datasets.

2. Clinical Applications of Radiomics and AI in Thymic Tumors:

Radiomics and AI have a wide range of clinical applications in thymic tumors:

a. Diagnosis:

- Radiomics can help differentiate thymic tumors from other mediastinal masses based on characteristic image features, improving accuracy in diagnosis.

b. Staging:

- Radiomics analysis can aid in precise staging by quantifying tumor size, shape, and invasion into adjacent structures, helping clinicians plan appropriate treatments.

c. Prognosis:

- Radiomics-based models can predict patient outcomes by assessing the aggressiveness of thymic tumors, the risk of recurrence, and overall survival.

d. Treatment Planning:

- Radiomics and AI assist in the delineation of tumor boundaries, optimizing radiation therapy planning, and helping surgeons plan precise tumor resections.

e. Treatment Response Monitoring:

- These technologies allow for real-time assessment of

treatment response by tracking changes in radiomic features before and after therapy.

f. Early Detection of Recurrence:

- Radiomics can detect minimal residual disease and early recurrence by identifying subtle changes in images that may precede clinical symptoms.

3. Recent Advancements in Radiomics and AI for Thymic Tumors:

Recent developments have propelled the use of radiomics and AI in thymic tumors:

a. Deep Learning Algorithms:

- Deep learning models, such as convolutional neural networks (CNNs), excel at feature extraction from images, enhancing the accuracy of radiomics-based predictions.

b. Multi-Modal Imaging Integration:

- Combining data from various imaging modalities, such as PET/CT and MRI, offers a more comprehensive view of thymic tumors.

c. Big Data and Cloud Computing:

- Access to large datasets and cloud-based computing infrastructure enables the development of robust AI models and facilitates real-time analysis.

d. Radiogenomics:

- Radiomics features can be correlated with genomic data to reveal associations between image patterns and genetic mutations, shedding light on tumor biology.

e. Explainable AI:

- Efforts are underway to make AI models more interpretable, enabling clinicians to understand the reasoning behind AI-generated recommendations.

f. Personalized Medicine:

- Radiomics and AI guide personalized treatment strategies by identifying patients who may benefit from targeted therapies or predicting individual responses to treatment.

4. Challenges and Considerations:

Despite their promise, radiomics and AI in thymic tumors face certain challenges:

a. Data Quality and Standardization:

- Ensuring the quality and standardization of imaging data is crucial for reliable radiomics and AI analysis.

b. Data Privacy and Security:

- The use of large datasets for AI raises concerns about patient privacy and data security.

c. Interpretability:

- Complex AI models may generate results that are difficult to interpret by clinicians, necessitating the development of explainable AI.

d. Clinical Validation:

- Radiomics and AI models need rigorous clinical validation to ensure their accuracy, reproducibility, and clinical utility.

e. Integration with Clinical Workflow:

- Seamless integration of radiomics and AI tools into the clinical workflow is essential for their adoption in routine practice.

f. Ethical and Legal Issues:

- Ethical considerations, such as bias in AI algorithms and liability in medical decision-making, require careful attention.

5. Future Directions:

The future of radiomics and AI in thymic tumors holds significant promise:

a. Early Detection and Prevention:

- AI models may enable the early detection of thymic tumors in high-risk individuals, potentially preventing disease progression.

b. Radiogenomic Correlations:

- Further integration of radiomics data with genomic information will provide a deeper understanding of the molecular underpinnings of thymic tumors.

c. Targeted Therapies:

- AI-driven patient stratification can identify candidates for targeted therapies, optimizing treatment outcomes.

d. Predictive Models:

- Advanced AI models will continue to improve the prediction of treatment response, recurrence risk, and long-term outcomes.

e. Real-time Decision Support:

- AI-based decision support systems will assist clinicians in real-time, enhancing diagnostic accuracy and treatment planning.

f. Population Health Management:

- AI can aid in population-level screening and management of thymic tumors, contributing to public health efforts.

6. Conclusion:

Radiomics and AI represent a transformative approach to thymic tumors, offering enhanced diagnostic accuracy, personalized treatment strategies, and real-time monitoring. Recent advancements in deep learning, multi-modal imaging, and radiogenomics are propelling these technologies to the forefront of thymic tumor care. While challenges such as data quality, interpretability, and clinical validation persist, ongoing research and innovation promise to further integrate radiomics and AI into routine clinical practice. These technologies hold the potential to improve patient outcomes, quality of life, and the overall management of thymic tumors, marking a significant step forward in the field of oncology.

9.5 Genomic Profiling for Personalized Medicine in Thymic Tumors: A Precision Approach to Treatment

Genomic profiling has emerged as a pivotal tool in the field of oncology, allowing for a personalized approach to cancer treatment. In the context of thymic tumors, a relatively rare and heterogeneous group of malignancies, genomic profiling holds great promise in guiding therapy decisions and improving patient outcomes. This section explores the principles of genomic profiling, its clinical applications, recent advancements, challenges, and the profound impact it has on personalized medicine in thymic tumors.

1. Genomic Profiling:

Genomic profiling, also known as molecular profiling or molecular diagnostics, involves the comprehensive analysis of an individual's tumor DNA, RNA, and proteins to identify genetic alterations and molecular markers specific to the cancer. This approach provides crucial insights into the biology of the tumor, its genetic drivers, and potential vulnerabilities that can be targeted with precision therapies.

2. Clinical Applications of Genomic Profiling in Thymic Tumors:

Genomic profiling plays a multifaceted role in thymic tumors:

a. Diagnosis and Subtyping:

- Identifying specific genetic alterations can aid in confirming the diagnosis and subclassifying thymic tumors, which can have different treatment approaches.

b. Treatment Selection:

- Genomic profiling helps determine the most appropriate treatment based on the presence of actionable mutations or biomarkers.

c. Predicting Treatment Response:

- Certain genetic alterations may predict the likelihood of responding to particular therapies, optimizing treatment choices.

d. Resistance Mechanisms:

- Monitoring genomic changes during treatment can reveal the emergence of resistance mechanisms, allowing for treatment adjustments.

e. Clinical Trials:

- Genomic profiling can identify eligible patients for clinical trials targeting specific genetic alterations or pathways.

3. Recent Advancements in Genomic Profiling for Thymic Tumors:

Recent developments have expanded the utility of genomic profiling in thymic tumors:

a. Next-Generation Sequencing (NGS):

- NGS technologies have enabled comprehensive analysis of the entire tumor genome, identifying mutations, copy number alterations, and structural variations.

b. Liquid Biopsies:

- Liquid biopsies, which analyze circulating tumor DNA (ctDNA), can provide real-time genomic information without the need for invasive procedures.

c. RNA Sequencing:

- RNA sequencing can reveal gene expression patterns and fusion genes, offering insights into tumor biology and potential therapeutic targets.

d. Proteomics:

- Proteomic profiling can identify protein biomarkers and assess protein expression levels, aiding in treatment decisions.

e. Multi-Omic Integration:

- Integrating data from genomics, transcriptomics, proteomics, and epigenomics provides a comprehensive view of the tumor's molecular landscape.

f. Targeted Therapies:

- Advances in targeted therapies, such as tyrosine kinase inhibitors and immunotherapies, have expanded the treatment options for patients with specific genomic alterations.

4. Challenges and Considerations:

Despite the promise of genomic profiling, several challenges must be addressed:

a. Tumor Heterogeneity:

- Tumors can display genetic heterogeneity, with different regions harboring distinct mutations. Obtaining a representative biopsy is crucial.

b. Actionable Targets:

- Not all identified genetic alterations have available targeted therapies, necessitating ongoing drug development efforts.

c. Resistance Mechanisms:

- Resistance to targeted therapies can develop over time due to acquired mutations or adaptive changes in the tumor.

d. Data Interpretation:

- Interpreting complex genomic data requires expertise

and infrastructure for data analysis and clinical decision support.

e. Cost and Accessibility:

- Genomic profiling can be expensive, and access may be limited in some healthcare settings.

5. Future Directions:

The future of genomic profiling in thymic tumors is promising:

a. Biomarker Discovery:

- Ongoing research will uncover new biomarkers and genetic alterations that provide deeper insights into thymic tumor biology.

b. Combination Therapies:

- Combinatorial approaches targeting multiple pathways or mutations may overcome resistance and improve treatment outcomes.

c. Liquid Biopsy Advancements:

- Liquid biopsies will continue to evolve, offering real-time monitoring and earlier detection of disease recurrence.

d. Genomic-Driven Clinical Trials:

- Clinical trials will increasingly incorporate genomic profiling to stratify patients and match them with targeted therapies.

e. Personalized Treatment Guidelines:

- Genomic profiling will lead to the development of personalized treatment guidelines for thymic tumors.

6. Conclusion:

Genomic profiling has ushered in a new era of personalized medicine in thymic tumors. By unraveling the genetic intricacies of these rare malignancies, clinicians can make informed treatment decisions, offering patients the best chance for a favorable outcome. Recent advancements in NGS, liquid biopsies, multi-omic integration, and targeted therapies have expanded the capabilities of genomic profiling. Despite challenges such as tumor heterogeneity and the need for actionable targets, ongoing research and clinical validation efforts are propelling this approach forward. As the field continues to evolve, genomic profiling will play an increasingly central role in the care of patients with thymic tumors, contributing to improved survival rates, enhanced quality of life, and a brighter outlook for those facing these complex malignancies.

9.6 Future Trends in Diagnostic Technologies for Thymic Tumors: Pioneering Advances on the Horizon

The landscape of diagnostic technologies for thymic tumors is on the brink of significant transformation, driven by innovative research, technological breakthroughs, and a growing understanding of tumor biology. In this section, we will explore the promising future trends that are poised to reshape the diagnosis and management of thymic tumors. These cutting-edge technologies hold the potential to enhance early detection, improve treatment outcomes, and elevate the quality of life for individuals affected by these rare malignancies.

1. Liquid Biopsies:

Advancing Sensitivity and Specificity

Liquid biopsies, which analyze circulating tumor DNA (ctDNA), circulating tumor cells (CTCs), and other biomolecules in bodily fluids, have already revolutionized cancer diagnostics. In the future, we can expect further improvements in the sensitivity and specificity of liquid biopsies for thymic tumors:

- **Ultra-sensitive Detection:** Novel techniques and assays will be developed to detect trace amounts of ctDNA or rare CTCs, enabling the diagnosis of thymic tumors at even earlier stages.
- **Multiplexed Analysis:** Liquid biopsies will evolve to simultaneously assess multiple genetic alterations, mutations, and protein markers, providing a comprehensive molecular profile of the tumor.
- **Epigenetic Markers:** Beyond genetic mutations, liquid biopsies will incorporate epigenetic markers, such as DNA methylation patterns, to enhance diagnostic accuracy and subtype classification.

2. Radiomics and AI:

Enhancing Predictive Modeling

The integration of radiomics and artificial intelligence (AI) is set to usher in a new era of diagnostic precision for thymic tumors. Future trends in this field include:

- **Real-time Decision Support:** AI algorithms will be seamlessly integrated into clinical workflows, providing radiologists and oncologists with real-time decision support for diagnosis, staging, and treatment planning.
- **Multimodal Fusion:** Radiomics will incorporate data from diverse imaging modalities, such as PET/CT, MRI, and functional imaging, to create more comprehensive

profiles of thymic tumors.
- **Deep Learning and Explainable AI:** Deep learning models will become more interpretable and capable of explaining their predictions, ensuring trust and transparency in clinical decision-making.
- **Quantitative Imaging Biomarkers:** Quantitative imaging biomarkers derived from radiomics will help predict treatment response, recurrence risk, and overall survival with greater accuracy.

3. Genomic Profiling:

Personalized Treatment Approaches

Genomic profiling will continue to play a central role in tailoring treatment strategies for thymic tumors:

- **Integration with Immunotherapy:** Genomic data will inform the selection of immunotherapies and the identification of patients likely to benefit from immune checkpoint inhibitors.
- **Combination Therapies:** Comprehensive genomic profiling will guide the development of combination therapies targeting multiple pathways and mutations, tackling treatment resistance more effectively.
- **Targeted Drug Development:** Insights from genomic profiling will drive the discovery of novel targeted therapies specifically designed for thymic tumors with unique genetic alterations.
- **Minimal Residual Disease Monitoring:** Genomic profiling will enable the sensitive detection of minimal residual disease, allowing for timely intervention in cases of recurrence.

4. Functional Imaging:

Unveiling Tumor Metabolism

Functional imaging techniques that assess tumor metabolism and microenvironment are poised to provide valuable insights into thymic tumors:

- **Metabolic Imaging:** Advances in PET imaging and other metabolic assessments will allow for the characterization of tumor metabolic profiles, aiding in diagnosis and treatment response monitoring.
- **Immunometabolism:** Functional imaging will help researchers understand the role of immunometabolism in thymic tumors and how it can be targeted for therapeutic benefit.

5. Artificial Intelligence in Pathology:

Transforming Histopathological Assessment

AI applications in pathology are set to revolutionize the interpretation of tissue samples from thymic tumors:

- **Digital Pathology:** Digital slide scanners and AI algorithms will automate the analysis of histopathological slides, reducing turnaround times and enhancing accuracy.
- **Molecular Pathology Integration:** AI will integrate molecular pathology data with histopathological findings, offering a comprehensive view of the tumor's biology.
- **Tumor Microenvironment Analysis:** AI will assess the tumor microenvironment, including immune cell infiltration and spatial organization, to predict treatment responses and prognosis.

6. Patient-Derived Organoids:

Personalized In Vitro Models

Patient-derived organoids, three-dimensional cultures of cells that mimic the structure and function of tumors, will play a pivotal role in drug testing and personalized medicine:

- **Drug Screening:** Thymic tumor organoids will be used to screen a wide range of therapies, helping identify the most effective treatments for individual patients.
- **Biomarker Discovery:** Organoids will aid in the discovery of novel biomarkers and genetic mutations that can guide treatment decisions.
- **Functional Studies:** Organoids will enable researchers to conduct functional studies of thymic tumors, unraveling their biology and therapeutic vulnerabilities.

7. Telemedicine and Remote Monitoring:

Improving Access to Specialized Care

Telemedicine and remote monitoring technologies will bridge geographical gaps, ensuring that patients with thymic tumors have access to specialized care and expert consultations:

- **Virtual Tumor Boards:** Multidisciplinary tumor boards will convene virtually, allowing experts from different locations to collaborate on treatment strategies.
- **Remote Monitoring Devices:** Wearable devices and remote monitoring tools will enable patients to track their health and treatment responses, providing real-time data to healthcare providers.
- **Telepathology:** Telepathology will enable pathologists to remotely assess histopathological samples, extending their expertise to underserved areas.

8. Patient Empowerment:

Informed Decision-Making

Empowering patients with information and support will be an integral part of future trends in thymic tumor diagnosis and management:

- **Patient Portals:** Comprehensive patient portals will provide individuals with access to their medical records, test results, and personalized treatment plans.
- **Genomic Counseling:** Genetic counselors will assist patients in understanding their genomic profiling results and the implications for treatment choices.
- **Supportive Apps:** Mobile applications will offer resources for symptom management, treatment tracking, and access to support networks.

9. Population-Level Screening:

Early Detection Initiatives

Public health initiatives will focus on early detection and prevention of thymic tumors:

- **High-Risk Populations:** Screening programs will target high-risk populations, such as individuals with specific genetic predispositions or prior radiation exposure.
- **Liquid Biopsy Screening:** Non-invasive liquid biopsies may become part of routine cancer screening, allowing for early detection of thymic tumors.
- **Public Awareness:** Educational campaigns will raise awareness of thymic tumors, their risk factors, and the importance of early diagnosis.

10. Multidisciplinary Collaboration:

Integrated Care Models

Collaboration among diverse healthcare professionals will be integral to improving thymic tumor care:

- **Tumor Board Integration:** Multidisciplinary tumor boards will become standard practice, ensuring that patients benefit from the expertise of oncologists, surgeons, radiologists, pathologists, and other specialists.
- **Research Consortia:** International research consortia will facilitate the sharing of data, samples, and insights, accelerating progress in thymic tumor research.

11. Ethical Considerations:

Balancing Innovation and Responsibility

As diagnostic technologies continue to advance, ethical considerations will remain paramount:

- **Data Privacy:** Ensuring the privacy and security of patients' genomic and medical data will be a critical ethical concern.
- **Equity and Access:** Efforts must be made to ensure that the benefits of cutting-edge diagnostics are accessible to all patients, regardless of socioeconomic status or geographical location.
- **Informed Consent:** Patients should be well-informed about the implications of genomic profiling, and informed consent processes should be transparent and comprehensive.

In conclusion, the future of diagnostic technologies for thymic tumors holds immense promise. From liquid biopsies and AI-enhanced radiomics to advanced genomic profiling and patient-derived organoids, these innovations are poised to enhance early detection, treatment selection, and monitoring. Moreover, telemedicine, patient empowerment, and population-level screening initiatives will democratize access to specialized care and promote early intervention. As these trends continue to evolve, multidisciplinary collaboration and ethical considerations will be central to ensuring that these technologies benefit patients while upholding the highest standards of care and responsibility. Thymic tumor diagnosis and management are on the cusp of transformative change, offering renewed hope and improved outcomes for individuals facing these challenging malignancies.

CHAPTER 10: TARGETED THERAPIES AND PRECISION MEDICINE

10.1 Molecular Targeting and Personalized Approaches in Thymic Tumors: A Precision Medicine Revolution

In the realm of thymic tumors, the era of one-size-fits-all treatment is gradually giving way to a more personalized and precise approach. Molecular targeting, driven by advancements in genomics and translational research, has become a cornerstone of thymic tumor management. This section delves into the pivotal role of molecular targeting, its clinical applications, recent breakthroughs, challenges, and the transformative impact it has on personalized medicine in the context of thymic tumors.

1. Molecular Targeting:

Molecular targeting, often referred to as precision medicine or targeted therapy, involves tailoring cancer treatment to the specific molecular alterations and pathways driving tumor growth. Unlike conventional chemotherapy, which indiscriminately targets rapidly dividing cells, molecular targeting aims to disrupt the molecular mechanisms that sustain cancer cells while sparing healthy tissue.

2. Clinical Applications of Molecular Targeting in Thymic Tumors:

Molecular targeting offers a spectrum of clinical applications in thymic tumors:

a. Targeted Therapies:

- Targeted therapies selectively inhibit specific proteins or pathways that are crucial for the survival and growth of thymic tumor cells.

b. Immunotherapies:

- Immunotherapies, such as immune checkpoint inhibitors, harness the patient's immune system to recognize and attack thymic tumor cells.

c. Combination Therapies:

- Combinatorial approaches involve the use of multiple targeted agents or targeted therapies in conjunction with other treatment modalities to achieve synergistic effects.

d. Personalized Treatment Plans:

- Molecular profiling informs treatment decisions by identifying actionable genetic alterations, allowing clinicians to tailor therapies to individual patients.

e. Predictive Biomarkers:

- Specific genetic alterations or biomarkers can predict treatment response, enabling the selection of the most effective therapy for each patient.

3. Recent Breakthroughs in Molecular Targeting for Thymic Tumors:

Recent developments in molecular targeting have expanded treatment options for thymic tumors:

a. Targeted Therapies:

- Tyrosine Kinase Inhibitors (TKIs): TKIs that target receptors such as EGFR and HER2 have shown promise in subsets of thymic tumors.
- mTOR Inhibitors: Drugs like everolimus target the mTOR pathway, which is frequently dysregulated in thymic tumors.

b. Immune Checkpoint Inhibitors:

- Immune checkpoint inhibitors, particularly PD-1 and PD-L1 inhibitors, have demonstrated efficacy in thymic tumors by unleashing the immune system to attack cancer cells.

c. Combination Strategies:

- Combining targeted therapies with immunotherapies or other agents is being explored to enhance treatment responses and overcome resistance.

d. Genomic Profiling:

- Comprehensive genomic profiling identifies specific mutations and genetic alterations that can be exploited as therapeutic targets.

e. Liquid Biopsies:

- Liquid biopsies are increasingly used to monitor treatment responses and identify emerging resistance mechanisms.

f. Preclinical Models:

- Patient-derived xenografts (PDX) and organoid models allow researchers to test potential targeted therapies in a preclinical setting.

4. Challenges and Considerations:

While molecular targeting holds great promise, several challenges must be navigated:

a. Resistance Mechanisms:

- Resistance to targeted therapies can develop over time, requiring ongoing research into resistance mechanisms and strategies to overcome them.

b. Biomarker Identification:

- Not all thymic tumors have well-defined molecular targets, necessitating the discovery of new biomarkers.

c. Access to Targeted Therapies:

- Ensuring equitable access to targeted therapies, especially for rare thymic tumor subtypes, is a critical consideration.

d. Combination Therapy Risks:

- The complexities of combining targeted therapies and immunotherapies must be carefully managed to avoid increased toxicities.

e. Immunotherapy Response Variability:

- Not all patients respond to immunotherapies, highlighting the need for predictive biomarkers of response.

5. Future Directions:

The future of molecular targeting in thymic tumors is poised for further advancements:

a. Expanded Targeted Therapies:

- The discovery of new molecular targets and the development of novel targeted therapies will expand treatment options.

b. Resistance Mitigation:

- Strategies to overcome resistance, such as second-line therapies and combination regimens, will be refined.

c. Immunotherapy Refinement:

- Research will focus on enhancing the efficacy of immunotherapies and identifying predictive markers of response.

d. Personalized Combinations:

- Tailored combinations of targeted therapies, immunotherapies, and conventional treatments will be explored for each patient.

e. Pediatric Population:

- Molecular targeting approaches will be adapted and optimized for pediatric thymic tumors, addressing unique challenges in this population.

f. Clinical Trials:

- Clinical trials will continue to investigate the safety and efficacy of emerging targeted therapies and combination strategies.

6. Conclusion:

Molecular targeting and personalized approaches represent a paradigm shift in thymic tumor management. By identifying the specific molecular drivers of each patient's tumor and tailoring treatments accordingly, clinicians can maximize therapeutic benefits while minimizing side effects. Recent breakthroughs in targeted therapies, immunotherapies, and genomics have expanded treatment options and improved patient outcomes. However, ongoing research is essential to address resistance mechanisms, refine combination strategies, and uncover new biomarkers. As molecular targeting continues to evolve, it holds the promise of transforming thymic tumor care, offering renewed hope to patients and the prospect of prolonged survival and an improved quality of life.

10.2 Emerging Therapeutic Targets in Thymic Tumors: Unlocking Novel Avenues for Treatment

The landscape of thymic tumors is undergoing a transformative shift, driven by ongoing research into emerging therapeutic targets. These targets, which encompass genetic, molecular, and immunological elements, hold the potential to revolutionize the treatment of thymic tumors. In this section, we will explore the exciting world of emerging therapeutic targets, their clinical implications, recent discoveries, challenges, and the promising impact they have on the future of thymic tumor therapy.

1. Emerging Therapeutic Targets:

Emerging therapeutic targets in thymic tumors encompass a diverse range of molecules and pathways that have shown potential as actionable elements for precision medicine. These targets hold the promise of more effective and targeted therapies, moving beyond the limitations of traditional treatment modalities.

2. Clinical Implications of Emerging Targets in Thymic

Tumors:

Emerging therapeutic targets have significant clinical implications for thymic tumors:

a. Targeted Therapies:

- Targeted therapies designed to inhibit or modulate specific emerging targets can offer more precise treatment options.

b. Immunotherapies:

- Emerging targets in the tumor microenvironment can be leveraged for immunotherapy development, enhancing the patient's immune response against the tumor.

c. Biomarker Discovery:

- Identifying and validating emerging targets can lead to the discovery of novel biomarkers for patient stratification and treatment response prediction.

d. Combination Therapies:

- Emerging targets can be incorporated into combination therapy approaches, increasing the chances of a favorable treatment response.

e. Personalized Medicine:

- Patient-specific molecular profiling can guide the selection of therapies targeting specific emerging targets, advancing the era of personalized medicine.

3. Recent Discoveries in Emerging Therapeutic Targets for Thymic Tumors:

Recent research efforts have uncovered a multitude of

emerging therapeutic targets in thymic tumors:

a. Genetic Alterations:

- Novel genetic alterations, such as mutations in the HRAS and NRAS genes, have been identified as potential targets for kinase inhibitors.

b. Immune Checkpoints:

- Beyond PD-1/PD-L1, emerging immune checkpoints like TIM-3, LAG-3, and TIGIT are being explored as targets for immunotherapy.

c. Tumor Microenvironment:

- Components of the tumor microenvironment, including tumor-associated macrophages and regulatory T cells, are being investigated as therapeutic targets.

d. Epigenetic Modifications:

- Epigenetic regulators like histone deacetylases (HDACs) and DNA methyltransferases are emerging targets for epigenetic therapy.

e. Vascular Targets:

- Angiogenesis inhibitors targeting VEGF and its receptors are being evaluated for their potential in thymic tumor treatment.

f. Novel Signaling Pathways:

- Emerging signaling pathways, such as the PI3K/Akt/mTOR pathway, are under investigation for targeted therapy development.

g. MicroRNAs:

- Dysregulated microRNAs in thymic tumors are being explored as potential targets or biomarkers for therapy.

4. Challenges and Considerations:

While the discovery of emerging therapeutic targets is promising, several challenges and considerations must be addressed:

a. Validation:

- Target validation is crucial to confirm the therapeutic relevance of emerging targets and assess their potential for clinical translation.

b. Resistance Mechanisms:

- Resistance to therapies targeting emerging targets can develop, necessitating strategies to overcome or prevent resistance.

c. Patient Stratification:

- Identifying which patients are most likely to benefit from therapies targeting emerging targets requires the development of predictive biomarkers.

d. Combination Therapy Risks:

- Combining therapies targeting multiple emerging targets may increase the risk of toxicities and side effects.

e. Pediatric Adaptation:

- Some emerging targets may require adaptation for use in pediatric thymic tumors, given the unique considerations of this population.

f. Clinical Trial Design:

- Designing clinical trials to assess the safety and efficacy of therapies targeting emerging targets requires careful planning and execution.

5. Future Directions:

The future of emerging therapeutic targets in thymic tumors is highly promising:

a. Precision Medicine:

- Advances in patient stratification based on emerging targets will enable more precise and effective treatment selection.

b. Combination Therapies:

- Combination therapies targeting multiple emerging targets and leveraging different treatment modalities will be explored to enhance treatment responses.

c. Resistance Mitigation:

- Strategies to overcome or prevent resistance to therapies targeting emerging targets will be a focus of research.

d. Pediatric Applications:

- Research into adapting emerging targets for pediatric thymic tumors will expand treatment options for young patients.

e. Early-Phase Trials:

- Early-phase clinical trials will continue to evaluate the safety and efficacy of therapies targeting emerging targets.

6. Conclusion:

Emerging therapeutic targets are ushering in a new era of hope and innovation in the management of thymic tumors. By unraveling the complex molecular and immunological landscape of these malignancies, researchers are identifying actionable elements that hold the potential to transform treatment paradigms. Recent discoveries in genetic alterations, immune checkpoints, the tumor microenvironment, and epigenetic modifications are expanding the toolkit for thymic tumor therapy. While challenges such as validation, resistance, and patient stratification persist, ongoing research and clinical trials are paving the way for more personalized and effective treatments. The future of thymic tumor management is increasingly defined by the promise of emerging therapeutic targets, offering patients the prospect of improved outcomes, extended survival, and an enhanced quality of life.

10.3 Immunotherapeutic Advancements in Thymic Tumors: Harnessing the Immune System for Precision Treatment

In recent years, immunotherapy has emerged as a groundbreaking approach in the treatment of various cancers, including thymic tumors. The immune system's ability to recognize and eliminate cancer cells has led to remarkable advancements in the field. This section explores the exciting developments in immunotherapeutic strategies for thymic tumors, their clinical applications, challenges, and the transformative impact they have on the management of these rare malignancies.

1. Immunotherapy:

Immunotherapy, also known as immune-based therapy, is a category of cancer treatment that harnesses the power of the immune system to target and destroy cancer cells. Unlike traditional treatments like chemotherapy, which directly attack cancer cells, immunotherapy enhances the body's natural defenses to recognize and eliminate cancer.

2. Clinical Applications of Immunotherapy in Thymic Tumors:

Immunotherapy has a range of clinical applications in thymic tumors:

a. Immune Checkpoint Inhibitors:

- Immune checkpoint inhibitors, such as PD-1/PD-L1 inhibitors, have demonstrated effectiveness in enhancing the immune system's ability to recognize and attack thymic tumor cells.

b. Adoptive Cell Therapy:

- Adoptive cell therapy involves the infusion of genetically modified or activated immune cells (such as CAR T-cells) to target thymic tumor cells.

c. Vaccines:

- Therapeutic cancer vaccines are designed to stimulate the immune system to recognize and target specific antigens present on thymic tumor cells.

d. Combination Therapies:

- Immunotherapy is often combined with other treatments, such as chemotherapy or radiation, to maximize treatment efficacy.

e. Maintenance Therapy:

- In some cases, immunotherapy is used as maintenance therapy to prevent disease recurrence.

f. Pediatric Applications:

- Immunotherapeutic approaches are adapted for pediatric thymic tumors, considering the unique characteristics of these cases.

3. Recent Developments in Immunotherapy for Thymic Tumors:

Recent research efforts have yielded significant advancements in immunotherapy for thymic tumors:

a. Immune Checkpoint Inhibitors:

- PD-1/PD-L1 inhibitors, such as pembrolizumab and nivolumab, have shown promising results in clinical trials for advanced thymic tumors.

b. Combination Therapies:

- Combinations of immune checkpoint inhibitors, or the addition of chemotherapy, are being explored to enhance response rates.

c. Biomarker Discovery:

- Efforts to identify predictive biomarkers, such as PD-L1 expression or tumor mutational burden, are ongoing to guide patient selection for immunotherapy.

d. CAR T-cell Therapy:

- CAR T-cell therapy is being investigated as a potential approach for thymic tumors, with early-phase clinical trials underway.

e. Vaccine Strategies:

- Research into therapeutic vaccines targeting specific antigens expressed by thymic tumors is advancing.

f. Pediatric Immunotherapy:

- Immunotherapeutic approaches are being adapted and studied in pediatric thymic tumors, offering new hope for young patients.

4. Challenges and Considerations:

Despite its promise, immunotherapy for thymic tumors presents several challenges and considerations:

a. Response Variability:

- Not all patients respond to immunotherapy, necessitating the identification of predictive biomarkers.

b. Resistance Mechanisms:

- Resistance to immunotherapy can develop, requiring research into strategies to overcome or prevent resistance.

c. Toxicities:

- Immune-related adverse events (irAEs) can occur as a result of immunotherapy and must be managed carefully.

d. Pediatric Considerations:

- Immunotherapy approaches for pediatric thymic tumors require special attention to potential long-term effects on young patients.

e. Combination Therapy Risks:

- The complexities of combining immunotherapy with other treatments must be carefully managed to avoid increased toxicities.

f. Patient Stratification:

- Developing methods for selecting the most appropriate patients for immunotherapy remains a challenge.

5. Future Directions:

The future of immunotherapy for thymic tumors is filled with promise:

a. Biomarker-Driven Treatment:

- Advancements in predictive biomarkers will enable more precise patient selection for immunotherapy.

b. Combination Strategies:

- The development of safe and effective combination therapies will be a focus of research.

c. Resistance Mitigation:

- Strategies to overcome or prevent resistance to immunotherapy will continue to evolve.

d. Pediatric Applications:

- Pediatric-specific immunotherapeutic approaches will be refined and expanded.

e. Clinical Trials:

- Ongoing and future clinical trials will explore the safety and efficacy of immunotherapies in thymic tumors.

6. Conclusion:

Immunotherapy has ushered in a new era of hope for individuals with thymic tumors. By harnessing the immune system's natural ability to recognize and eliminate cancer cells, researchers and clinicians are transforming the treatment landscape for these rare malignancies. Recent developments in immune checkpoint inhibitors, adoptive cell therapy, vaccines, and combination therapies have shown promising results. While challenges such as response variability, resistance, and toxicities persist, ongoing research and clinical trials are driving progress. The future of thymic tumor management is increasingly defined by the potential of immunotherapy, offering patients the prospect of improved outcomes, prolonged survival, and a better quality of life.

10.4 Resistance Mechanisms and Overcoming Challenges in Thymic Tumor Immunotherapy

Immunotherapy has revolutionized the treatment of various cancers, including thymic tumors. However, as with any cancer treatment, the development of resistance poses a significant challenge. This section explores the resistance mechanisms encountered in thymic tumor immunotherapy, strategies to overcome these challenges, and the ongoing research efforts to enhance the effectiveness of these groundbreaking therapies.

1. Resistance Mechanisms in Immunotherapy:

Resistance to immunotherapy occurs when cancer cells adapt and evade the immune system's attack. Understanding the underlying mechanisms is crucial to improving treatment outcomes in thymic tumors.

2. Mechanisms of Resistance:

Several mechanisms contribute to resistance in thymic tumor immunotherapy:

a. Immune Checkpoint Overexpression:

- Upregulation of immune checkpoint molecules like PD-L1 on cancer cells can inhibit immune cell activity, reducing the effectiveness of checkpoint inhibitors.

b. Tumor Microenvironment Alterations:

- Changes in the tumor microenvironment, such as increased infiltration of suppressive immune cells (Tregs, myeloid-derived suppressor cells) or reduced T-cell infiltration, can promote immune evasion.

c. Antigen Loss or Heterogeneity:

- Cancer cells may downregulate target antigens recognized by immune cells, rendering them less susceptible to attack.

d. Immune Exclusion:

- Tumors can develop physical barriers, like a dense extracellular matrix, preventing immune cell infiltration.

e. Tumor-Induced Immunosuppression:

- The secretion of immunosuppressive cytokines, such as TGF-β or IL-10, by tumor cells can inhibit immune cell function.

f. Genetic Alterations:

- Mutations in genes related to antigen presentation, interferon signaling, or the antigen-processing machinery can hinder immune recognition.

g. Exhausted T-cells:

- Prolonged exposure to tumor antigens and immune checkpoints can exhaust T-cells, reducing their ability to mount an effective response.

3. Overcoming Resistance Mechanisms:

Addressing resistance mechanisms is vital to improving the efficacy of thymic tumor immunotherapy:

a. Combination Therapies:

- Combining immunotherapies with other agents, such as chemotherapy or targeted therapies, can overcome resistance by attacking cancer cells through multiple mechanisms.

b. Immune Checkpoint Inhibitor Combinations:

- Combining PD-1/PD-L1 inhibitors with other checkpoint inhibitors, like CTLA-4 inhibitors, can enhance immune responses.

c. Targeted Therapies:

- Targeted therapies, such as tyrosine kinase inhibitors or mTOR inhibitors, may be used in combination with immunotherapy to target specific pathways driving resistance.

d. Adaptive Therapy:

- Adaptive therapy strategies involve alternating treatment intensity to maintain tumor control while minimizing resistance.

e. Biomarker-Guided Treatment:

- Identifying predictive biomarkers for treatment response can help select patients who are more likely to benefit from immunotherapy.

f. Overcoming Immune Exclusion:

- Strategies to break down physical barriers in the tumor microenvironment, such as using matrix-modifying agents, may improve immune cell infiltration.

g. Immunomodulatory Agents:

- Agents that modulate the immune system, such as interferon or immune stimulants, can be used in combination with immunotherapy.

h. Epigenetic Modulators:

- Epigenetic therapies may reprogram immune cells to enhance their anti-tumor activity.

4. Ongoing Research Efforts:

Continued research is crucial for understanding and overcoming resistance in thymic tumor immunotherapy:

a. Resistance Mechanism Discovery:

- Ongoing research aims to identify novel resistance mechanisms, allowing for targeted therapeutic approaches.

b. Combination Trials:

- Clinical trials evaluating various combination therapies are ongoing to assess their efficacy and safety in thymic tumors.

c. Biomarker Discovery:

- Identifying robust predictive biomarkers for immunotherapy response remains a priority.

d. Immunotherapy Sequencing:

- Studies are exploring the optimal sequencing of immunotherapy with other treatment modalities.

e. Pediatric Considerations:

- Research into resistance mechanisms in pediatric thymic tumors and the development of age-appropriate strategies are ongoing.

f. Early Detection of Resistance:

- Developing methods to detect resistance early in the treatment course can guide timely interventions.

5. Challenges and Considerations:

Overcoming resistance in thymic tumor immunotherapy is not without its challenges:

a. Individual Variability:

- Resistance mechanisms may vary from patient to patient, necessitating personalized approaches.

b. Toxicity Management:

- Combining therapies can increase the risk of toxicities, requiring careful management.

c. Data Collection:

- Comprehensive data collection and analysis are essential for understanding resistance mechanisms and treatment outcomes.

d. Clinical Trial Access:

- Access to clinical trials exploring novel combinations or therapies may be limited for some patients.

e. Pediatric-Specific Challenges:

- Pediatric patients may face unique resistance mechanisms and require tailored strategies.

6. Conclusion:

Resistance mechanisms represent a formidable challenge in thymic tumor immunotherapy. However, ongoing research efforts, combination therapies, and the identification of predictive biomarkers offer hope for overcoming these obstacles. By understanding and addressing resistance mechanisms, clinicians can enhance the effectiveness of immunotherapy, extending the lives of individuals with thymic tumors and improving their quality of life. As research continues to uncover the intricacies of resistance, thymic tumor treatment is poised to evolve, offering new opportunities for personalized, effective, and lasting therapies.

10.5 Adverse Events and Management in Thymic Tumor Immunotherapy

Immunotherapy has revolutionized the treatment of thymic tumors, offering new hope and improved outcomes for patients. However, like all medical interventions, immunotherapy can be associated with adverse events or side effects. This section explores the spectrum of adverse events related to thymic tumor immunotherapy, their management, strategies for prevention, and the importance of patient and healthcare provider communication in optimizing treatment outcomes.

1. Adverse Events in Immunotherapy:

Adverse events, often referred to as side effects or toxicities, are undesirable and unintended effects of medical treatments. In thymic tumor immunotherapy, adverse events can vary in severity and may impact patients' quality of life.

2. Types of Adverse Events in Immunotherapy:

Adverse events associated with immunotherapy for thymic tumors can affect various organ systems:

a. Immune-Related Adverse Events (irAEs):

- IrAEs are a hallmark of immunotherapy and can affect virtually any organ. Common irAEs include skin rashes, colitis, pneumonitis, hepatitis, and endocrine abnormalities.

b. Infusion-Related Reactions:

- Infusion-related reactions, such as fever, chills, and allergic responses, can occur during or shortly after immunotherapy administration.

c. Hematological Adverse Events:

- Some immunotherapies can lead to changes in blood cell counts, such as anemia, neutropenia, or thrombocytopenia.

d. Dermatological Adverse Events:

- Skin-related side effects, including rashes, pruritus (itching), and skin inflammation, are common.

e. Gastrointestinal Adverse Events:

- Diarrhea, nausea, vomiting, and colitis can affect the digestive system.

f. Endocrine Adverse Events:

- Hormone imbalances, such as thyroid dysfunction or adrenal insufficiency, can occur.

g. Cardiac Adverse Events:

- In rare cases, immunotherapy may lead to cardiac complications, such as myocarditis.

h. Neurological Adverse Events:

- Neurological side effects, including neuropathy or cognitive changes, are infrequent but important to monitor.

i. Pulmonary Adverse Events:

- Pneumonitis, a potentially serious lung condition, can develop as a result of immunotherapy.

3. Severity Grading of Adverse Events:

To facilitate communication between healthcare providers and patients, adverse events are often categorized based on their severity using grading systems like the Common Terminology Criteria for Adverse Events (CTCAE). Grades range from mild (Grade 1) to life-threatening (Grade 5).

4. Management of Adverse Events:

Effectively managing adverse events is critical to ensuring the safety and tolerability of immunotherapy. Strategies for management include:

a. Early Detection:

- Prompt recognition of adverse events is essential. Patients should be educated on potential side effects and encouraged to report any symptoms to their healthcare team.

b. Grading and Monitoring:

- Healthcare providers use grading systems to assess the severity of adverse events. Frequent monitoring and follow-up appointments help track changes in symptoms.

c. Treatment Modifications:

- Depending on the severity of adverse events, treatment

may need to be temporarily or permanently halted. Dose reductions or delays can also be considered.

d. Symptomatic Relief:

- Medications and interventions can be prescribed to alleviate specific symptoms, such as anti-inflammatory drugs for colitis or steroids for immune-related adverse events.

e. Specialist Consultations:

- In cases of severe or complex adverse events, specialists in relevant fields, such as dermatology, cardiology, or neurology, may be consulted.

f. Supportive Care:

- Supportive measures, such as hydration, pain management, and nutritional support, can help patients cope with side effects.

5. Prevention of Adverse Events:

While not all adverse events can be prevented, several strategies can minimize their occurrence:

a. Patient Education:

- Thoroughly educating patients about the potential side effects of immunotherapy and the importance of reporting symptoms promptly is crucial.

b. Risk Assessment:

- Healthcare providers may assess patients' risk factors, such as preexisting conditions, to tailor treatment plans accordingly.

c. Monitoring Protocols:

- Implementing regular monitoring protocols during treatment can help detect adverse events early.

d. Personalized Treatment Plans:

- Tailoring immunotherapy regimens to individual patients' needs and tolerability can reduce the risk of severe side effects.

e. Supportive Measures:

- Providing patients with access to supportive care services, such as nutrition counseling or psychological support, can improve their overall well-being during treatment.

6. Communication and Shared Decision-Making:

Effective communication between patients and healthcare providers is paramount:

a. Informed Consent:

- Patients should be well-informed about the potential risks and benefits of immunotherapy and provide informed consent before starting treatment.

b. Open Dialogue:

- Patients are encouraged to discuss any concerns or questions they have with their healthcare team, fostering a collaborative and transparent relationship.

c. Shared Decision-Making:

- Shared decision-making involves patients actively participating in treatment decisions, considering their values and preferences alongside medical expertise.

d. Reporting Adverse Events:

- Patients should promptly report any symptoms or adverse events to their healthcare providers to enable early intervention.

7. Challenges and Considerations:

The management of adverse events in thymic tumor immunotherapy presents challenges:

a. Individual Variation:

- Adverse event profiles can vary significantly among patients, making tailored approaches necessary.

b. Rare but Serious Events:

- While severe adverse events are relatively rare, they can have serious consequences, underscoring the importance of vigilant monitoring.

c. Pediatric-Specific Considerations:

- Managing adverse events in pediatric thymic tumor patients requires specialized knowledge and age-appropriate care.

d. Psychological Impact:

- Adverse events can have a psychological impact on patients, and addressing their emotional well-being is an essential component of comprehensive care.

8. Conclusion:

Adverse events are an inherent part of immunotherapy for thymic tumors. However, with vigilant monitoring, early detection, tailored management, and open communication between patients and healthcare providers, the impact of adverse events can be minimized. Patient safety and well-being remain the top priorities in the evolving landscape of thymic tumor treatment, where immunotherapy continues to offer hope and improved outcomes for individuals facing this rare malignancy.

10.6 The Future of Precision Medicine in Thymic Tumors: Unlocking Personalized Treatment Approaches

As the field of oncology advances, precision medicine is emerging as a transformative approach to the treatment of thymic tumors. Precision medicine tailors treatment strategies to the unique genetic, molecular, and immunological characteristics of individual patients and their tumors. In this section, we explore the promising future of precision medicine in thymic tumors, including the role of genomics, targeted therapies, immunotherapy, and the integration of multidisciplinary care for improved patient outcomes.

1. Precision Medicine:

Precision medicine, also known as personalized medicine, is a paradigm shift in healthcare that recognizes the individuality of each patient's disease. Instead of a one-size-fits-all approach, precision medicine aims to deliver the right treatment to the right patient at the right time.

2. Genomic Profiling:

Genomic profiling, the analysis of a patient's genetic makeup, is at the forefront of precision medicine for thymic tumors:

a. Tumor Genomics:

- Comprehensive genomic sequencing of thymic tumors can identify mutations, amplifications, and fusions that drive tumor growth. This information guides treatment selection and clinical trial eligibility.

b. Germline Genetic Testing:

- Identifying germline mutations in genes associated with thymic tumors, such as those in familial syndromes, informs screening and preventive strategies for at-risk individuals.

c. Predictive Biomarkers:

- Genomic profiling helps identify predictive biomarkers for immunotherapy, targeted therapies, and chemotherapy responses.

d. Resistance Mechanisms:

- Understanding genomic alterations associated with treatment resistance enables the development of strategies to overcome resistance.

3. Targeted Therapies:

Targeted therapies focus on specific molecular targets within thymic tumors:

a. EGFR Inhibitors:

- Epidermal growth factor receptor (EGFR) inhibitors, such as erlotinib, are being explored for tumors with EGFR mutations.

b. Kinase Inhibitors:

- Tyrosine kinase inhibitors (TKIs), including sunitinib and pazopanib, may have utility in tumors with activated kinase pathways.

c. Immune Checkpoint Inhibitors:

- Precision medicine identifies patients who are most likely to benefit from immune checkpoint inhibitors based on biomarker expression.

d. PARP Inhibitors:

- Poly (ADP-ribose) polymerase (PARP) inhibitors are being investigated in tumors with DNA repair pathway mutations.

e. mTOR Inhibitors:

- mTOR inhibitors like everolimus have shown promise in thymic tumors with mTOR pathway activation.

f. HER2 Targeting:

- HER2-targeted therapies are explored in tumors with HER2 amplifications.

4. Immunotherapy Personalization:

Immunotherapy is a cornerstone of precision medicine for thymic tumors:

a. Predictive Biomarkers:

- Identifying biomarkers like PD-L1 expression or tumor mutational burden helps select patients who are more likely to respond to immune checkpoint inhibitors.

b. Combination Strategies:

- Combining immunotherapy with targeted therapies or other immune-modulating agents is a personalized approach to enhance treatment efficacy.

c. CAR T-cell Therapy:

- Chimeric antigen receptor (CAR) T-cell therapy can be tailored to target specific antigens expressed on thymic tumor cells.

5. Liquid Biopsies:

Liquid biopsies involve analyzing tumor-related genetic material (e.g., ctDNA) from a patient's blood:

a. Non-Invasive Monitoring:

- Liquid biopsies offer a non-invasive method to monitor tumor dynamics, detect resistance mechanisms, and assess treatment response.

b. Early Detection:

- Detecting minimal residual disease or recurrence early through liquid biopsies allows for timely intervention.

6. Radiomics and AI:

Radiomics, the extraction of quantitative features from medical images, combined with artificial intelligence (AI) algorithms, is revolutionizing thymic tumor diagnosis and treatment:

a. Predictive Modeling:

- AI models can predict treatment response, overall survival, and recurrence risk based on radiomic features.

b. Treatment Planning:

- Radiomics aids in treatment planning by providing insights into tumor heterogeneity and biology.

c. Image-Guided Interventions:

- AI-enhanced image analysis facilitates precise tumor localization during radiation therapy and surgery.

7. Multidisciplinary Care:

Multidisciplinary teams, including oncologists, surgeons, radiologists, pathologists, and genetic counselors, collaborate to tailor precision medicine strategies for thymic tumors:

a. Comprehensive Evaluation:

- Multidisciplinary evaluation ensures a comprehensive understanding of the patient's disease and treatment options.

b. Treatment Sequencing:

- Coordination between specialists helps determine the optimal sequencing of surgery, radiation therapy, and systemic treatments.

c. Clinical Trials:

- Multidisciplinary teams play a crucial role in identifying and enrolling eligible patients in clinical trials of novel precision therapies.

8. Pediatric Considerations:

Precision medicine in pediatric thymic tumors demands specialized approaches:

a. Germline Testing:

- Germline testing identifies genetic predispositions, guiding risk assessment and family counseling.

b. Targeted Therapies:

- Pediatric-specific targeted therapies are explored to address the unique molecular characteristics of young patients.

c. Survivorship Care:

- Long-term follow-up and monitoring are vital for addressing late effects and ensuring the well-being of pediatric survivors.

9. Ethical and Social Implications:

Precision medicine raises ethical considerations, including data privacy, informed consent, and equitable access to advanced treatments:

a. Informed Decision-Making:

- Patients and families must understand the potential benefits, risks, and uncertainties of precision medicine options.

b. Data Security:

- Protecting patient genetic and health data is paramount to maintain trust in precision medicine.

c. Health Equity:

- Efforts are needed to ensure that all patients, regardless of socioeconomic status or geographic location, have equitable access to precision treatments.

10. Challenges and Considerations:

Despite the promise of precision medicine, challenges remain:

a. Tumor Heterogeneity:

- Thymic tumors exhibit significant heterogeneity, necessitating comprehensive profiling for accurate treatment selection.

b. Rarity of Thymic Tumors:

- The rarity of thymic tumors poses challenges in conducting large-scale clinical trials and developing targeted therapies.

c. Resistance Mechanisms:

- Identifying and overcoming resistance mechanisms in precision treatments is an ongoing challenge.

d. Pediatric-Specific Challenges:

- Adapting precision approaches for pediatric thymic tumors requires specialized expertise and infrastructure.

11. Conclusion:

The future of precision medicine in thymic tumors holds great promise for improving patient outcomes. By harnessing genomics, targeted therapies, immunotherapy, liquid biopsies, radiomics, and multidisciplinary care, precision medicine allows for tailored treatment strategies that address the individual characteristics of each patient and their tumor. As research and technology continue to advance, the integration of precision medicine into thymic tumor management offers hope for more effective therapies, prolonged survival, and enhanced quality of life for individuals facing these rare malignancies.

CHAPTER 11: EXPERIMENTAL MODELS AND BASIC RESEARCH

11.1 Animal Models of Thymic Tumorigenesis: Insights into Disease Mechanisms and Therapeutic Development

Animal models play a crucial role in advancing our understanding of thymic tumorigenesis, from elucidating disease mechanisms to evaluating potential therapeutic interventions. This section delves into the diverse range of animal models used to study thymic tumors, highlighting their contributions to research, insights gained, and their relevance in developing novel treatment strategies for this rare and complex malignancy.

1. Animal Models in Thymic Tumorigenesis:

Animal models are invaluable tools for studying the biology, pathogenesis, and treatment of human diseases. In the context of thymic tumors, animal models have provided critical insights into disease development and progression, as well as serving as platforms for preclinical testing of therapeutic interventions.

2. Murine Models:

Murine models, particularly mice, have been widely used in thymic tumor research due to their genetic similarity to humans and the availability of genetically engineered strains:

a. Spontaneous Models:

- Spontaneous thymic tumors can develop in certain mouse strains, such as the AKR/J or p53-deficient strains. These models mimic the natural course of tumorigenesis and offer insights into genetic predispositions.

b. Genetically Engineered Models (GEMs):

- GEMs, including transgenic and knockout mice, allow researchers to manipulate specific genes implicated in thymic tumorigenesis. For example, the K5-mTert model exhibits telomerase activation, which is a common event in thymic tumors.

c. Xenograft Models:

- Human thymic tumor cells can be xenografted into immunocompromised mice, providing a platform for testing potential therapeutics and evaluating tumor behavior in vivo.

d. Patient-Derived Xenografts (PDXs):

- PDX models involve implanting patient-derived tumor tissue into immunodeficient mice. These models better capture the heterogeneity and biology of human thymic tumors and are valuable for drug screening.

3. Zebrafish Models:

Zebrafish models have gained popularity in cancer research due to their rapid development, transparency, and genetic tractability:

a. Transgenic Zebrafish:

- Transgenic zebrafish lines can be engineered to express oncogenes or tumor suppressor genes relevant to thymic tumors. These models allow for real-time visualization of tumorigenesis.

b. Xenotransplantation:

- Human thymic tumor cells can be transplanted into zebrafish embryos or adult zebrafish, enabling the assessment of tumor growth and metastasis.

4. Avian Models:

Avian models, such as quails and chickens, have been used to study the development of the thymus and thymic tumors:

a. Avian Embryos:

- Chick embryos provide a unique system for investigating thymus development and the role of specific genes in thymic tumorigenesis.

5. Canine Models:

Canine models offer translational relevance, as dogs naturally develop thymic tumors that share similarities with those in humans:

a. Canine Spontaneous Models:

- Certain dog breeds, like Cavalier King Charles Spaniels and Fox Terriers, are predisposed to thymic tumors. Studying these cases can provide insights into genetic predispositions.

b. Clinical Trials:

- Canine clinical trials for thymic tumors can evaluate

the safety and efficacy of therapies, benefiting both dogs and humans.

6. Insights Gained from Animal Models:

Animal models of thymic tumorigenesis have yielded valuable insights:

a. Genetic Determinants:

- GEMs have identified key genetic alterations driving thymic tumor formation, such as mutations in genes like p53, KIT, and EGFR.

b. Immune Microenvironment:

- Animal models have elucidated the role of the immune microenvironment in thymic tumors, informing immunotherapy strategies.

c. Metastasis:

- Xenograft and zebrafish models have shed light on the metastatic potential of thymic tumors and mechanisms underlying their spread.

d. Therapeutic Testing:

- Animal models have served as preclinical platforms for testing novel therapeutics, including targeted agents and immunotherapies.

e. Early Detection:

- Zebrafish and avian models have contributed to the understanding of early thymus development and potential interventions at this stage.

7. Challenges and Limitations:

Despite their advantages, animal models have limitations:

a. Species Differences:

- Variations between species can limit the direct applicability of findings to humans, necessitating caution in extrapolating results.

b. Complex Biology:

- Thymic tumors are biologically diverse, and models may not fully recapitulate this complexity.

c. Ethical and Practical Considerations:

- Ethical concerns and logistical challenges can arise in maintaining and conducting experiments with animal models.

8. Future Directions:

The future of animal models in thymic tumorigenesis research holds promise:

a. Advanced Genetic Models:

- Continued development of genetically engineered mouse models that better mimic human thymic tumors is anticipated.

b. Xenotransplantation:

- Improved patient-derived xenograft models are expected to enhance preclinical drug testing and personalized medicine approaches.

c. Integration of Technologies:

- Combining animal models with cutting-edge technologies like CRISPR-Cas9 editing and single-cell RNA sequencing will deepen our understanding of thymic tumor biology.

d. Comparative Oncology:

- Expanding comparative oncology studies in dogs may reveal novel therapeutic strategies.

e. Ethical Considerations:

- Ethical frameworks for animal research will continue to evolve, emphasizing humane practices and minimizing harm.

9. Conclusion:

Animal models of thymic tumorigenesis have been invaluable in advancing our understanding of this rare malignancy. They have provided insights into disease mechanisms, allowed for preclinical testing of therapies, and paved the way for personalized treatment approaches. As research continues to evolve, these models will remain essential tools in the quest to improve outcomes for individuals with thymic tumors, offering hope for more effective treatments and, ultimately, a cure.

11.2 Cell Culture Systems and In Vitro Studies in Thymic Tumorigenesis

Cell culture systems and in vitro studies are indispensable tools in thymic tumorigenesis research. These approaches provide controlled environments to investigate various aspects of thymic tumors, including their biology, genetics, signaling pathways, drug responses, and potential therapeutic targets. This section delves into the significance of cell culture systems and in vitro studies in advancing our understanding of thymic tumors and the development of novel treatment strategies.

1. In Vitro Studies:

In vitro studies involve the cultivation of thymic tumor cells or relevant cell types in controlled laboratory conditions. These studies offer several advantages, including the ability to dissect specific cellular processes, evaluate drug responses, and conduct high-throughput experiments.

2. Establishment of Thymic Tumor Cell Lines:

The establishment of thymic tumor cell lines has been pivotal in studying the biology and genetics of these rare malignancies:

a. Primary Tumor Samples:

- Thymic tumor cell lines are often derived from primary tumor samples obtained from patients through biopsies or surgical resections.

b. Immortalization Techniques:

- Immortalization methods, such as introducing telomerase or oncogenes, can facilitate the long-term growth of primary cells.

c. Authentication and Characterization:

- Proper authentication and characterization of cell lines are crucial to ensure their relevance and reliability in research.

3. Types of In Vitro Studies:

In vitro studies encompass a broad range of investigations in thymic tumorigenesis:

a. Cell Proliferation and Viability:

- Assessing the growth and viability of thymic tumor cells under different conditions and treatments.

b. Genetic and Molecular Profiling:

- Analyzing the genetic and molecular characteristics of thymic tumor cells using techniques like PCR, Western blotting, and next-generation sequencing.

c. Signaling Pathway Analysis:

- Investigating the activation or inhibition of specific signaling pathways within thymic tumor cells.

d. Drug Screening and Sensitivity Testing:

- Evaluating the response of thymic tumor cells to various drugs, including chemotherapeutic agents, targeted therapies, and immunotherapies.

e. 3D Culture Models:

- Developing three-dimensional culture models to better mimic the tumor microenvironment and assess drug responses.

f. Co-Culture Systems:

- Studying interactions between thymic tumor cells and immune cells, fibroblasts, or other stromal components.

g. CRISPR-Cas9 Gene Editing:

- Using gene-editing techniques to manipulate specific genes within thymic tumor cells and study their functional roles.

4. Insights Gained from In Vitro Studies:

In vitro studies have yielded critical insights into thymic tumorigenesis:

a. Genetic Alterations:

- Identification of key genetic alterations, including mutations in genes like p53, KIT, and EGFR, that drive thymic tumor development.

b. Signaling Pathways:

- Elucidation of dysregulated signaling pathways, such as the PI3K/AKT/mTOR pathway, providing potential targets for therapy.

c. Drug Sensitivity:

- Assessment of drug sensitivity profiles, enabling the identification of potential therapeutic agents and combinations.

d. Immunotherapy Targets:

- Identification of immune checkpoint molecules and tumor-associated antigens that can be targeted with immunotherapy.

e. Resistance Mechanisms:

- Understanding mechanisms of drug resistance, informing strategies to overcome treatment challenges.

f. Biomarker Discovery:

- Discovery of potential biomarkers for prognosis, patient stratification, and treatment response prediction.

5. Challenges and Considerations:

In vitro studies have limitations and challenges:

a. Simplified Models:

- In vitro systems lack the complexity of the tumor microenvironment, potentially limiting the relevance of findings.

b. Genetic Drift:

- Long-term culture of cell lines can lead to genetic changes that may not reflect the original tumor.

c. Translational Gap:

- Findings from in vitro studies must be validated in preclinical animal models and clinical trials.

d. Ethical Use of Resources:

- Proper ethical considerations and resource management are essential in cell line establishment and experiments.

6. Advanced Techniques in In Vitro Studies:

Advancements in techniques further enhance the utility of in vitro studies:

a. Organoids:

- Thymic tumor organoids, three-dimensional miniaturized organs grown from tumor cells, more accurately mimic the in vivo tumor microenvironment.

b. Microfluidic Devices:

- Microfluidic platforms enable precise control over cellular microenvironments, facilitating studies of cell-cell interactions and drug responses.

c. High-Throughput Screening:

- Automated high-throughput screening assays allow the rapid testing of numerous drug candidates against thymic tumor cells.

d. Multi-Omics Integration:

- Integrating genomics, transcriptomics, proteomics, and metabolomics data provides a holistic view of thymic tumor biology.

7. Personalized Medicine Approaches:

In vitro studies are integral to personalized medicine approaches for thymic tumors:

a. Patient-Derived Models:

- Patient-derived cell lines and organoids enable the screening of individualized treatment options.

b. Drug Testing Platforms:

- High-throughput drug testing platforms help identify the most effective treatments for specific patient profiles.

c. Biomarker Validation:

- In vitro studies validate potential biomarkers for predicting treatment responses in individual patients.

8. Future Directions:

The future of in vitro studies in thymic tumorigenesis research holds significant promise:

a. Improved Organoid Models:

- The development of more advanced thymic tumor organoid models will better mimic the in vivo tumor microenvironment.

b. High-Throughput Technologies:

- Continued advancements in high-throughput technologies will expedite drug discovery and validation.

c. Integration with Clinical Data:

- Integrating in vitro findings with clinical data will enhance our ability to tailor treatments to individual patients.

d. Ethics and Reproducibility:

- Ethical considerations and rigorous experimental design will continue to be paramount.

9. Conclusion:

In vitro studies and cell culture systems are invaluable tools in advancing our understanding of thymic tumors. They provide controlled environments for dissecting the biology of these malignancies, identifying potential therapeutic targets, and evaluating drug responses. As technology and techniques evolve, in vitro studies will play an increasingly vital role in developing personalized treatment strategies for thymic tumors, ultimately improving patient outcomes and quality of life.

11.3 Insights from Genomic and Proteomic Research in Thymic Tumorigenesis

Genomic and proteomic research has revolutionized our understanding of thymic tumorigenesis by unraveling the intricate molecular mechanisms underlying the development and progression of these rare malignancies. This section delves into the significance of genomic and proteomic research in shedding light on thymic tumors, identifying potential therapeutic targets, and paving the way for precision medicine approaches.

1. Genomic and Proteomic Research:

Genomic research focuses on the study of an organism's complete set of genes (genome), while proteomic research investigates the entire complement of proteins (proteome) expressed by an organism. In the context of thymic tumorigenesis, these approaches have been instrumental in deciphering the molecular complexities of these rare tumors.

2. Genomic Alterations in Thymic Tumors:

Understanding the genomic alterations in thymic tumors has been a pivotal aspect of research:

a. Mutations:

- Comprehensive genomic sequencing has revealed mutations in key genes such as TP53, KIT, EGFR, and HRAS. These mutations contribute to tumorigenesis and provide potential targets for therapy.

b. Copy Number Alterations:

- Genomic studies have identified copy number alterations, including amplifications and deletions, that impact critical oncogenes and tumor suppressor genes.

c. Telomere Maintenance Mechanisms:

- Investigations into telomere maintenance mechanisms, such as telomerase activation, have illuminated the role of telomeres in thymic tumorigenesis.

d. Chromosomal Rearrangements:

- Chromosomal rearrangements, such as the t(15;19)

translocation resulting in CIC-DUX4 fusion, have been identified in subsets of thymic tumors.

3. Molecular Subtypes:

Genomic research has led to the classification of thymic tumors into distinct molecular subtypes:

a. Type A, AB, B1, B2, and B3 Thymomas:

- Each subtype exhibits specific genomic alterations, reflecting differences in biological behavior and potential therapeutic targets.

b. Thymic Carcinomas:

- Genomic studies have highlighted the genetic heterogeneity of thymic carcinomas, underscoring the need for personalized treatment strategies.

4. Proteomic Profiling:

Proteomic research has focused on identifying proteins associated with thymic tumorigenesis:

a. Biomarker Discovery:

- Proteomic studies have uncovered potential biomarkers for early detection, prognosis, and treatment response prediction.

b. Signaling Pathways:

- Proteomic analyses have elucidated dysregulated signaling pathways, including the PI3K/AKT/mTOR pathway, that are critical in thymic tumorigenesis.

c. Immune Microenvironment:

- Characterizing the proteome of the immune microenvironment in thymic tumors has provided insights into immune evasion mechanisms and potential targets for immunotherapy.

5. Precision Medicine Approaches:

Genomic and proteomic research has paved the way for precision medicine approaches in thymic tumorigenesis:

a. Targeted Therapies:

- Identifying specific genomic alterations has enabled the development of targeted therapies, such as EGFR inhibitors and mTOR inhibitors.

b. Immunotherapy:

- Proteomic profiling of the immune microenvironment has informed the use of immune checkpoint inhibitors and CAR T-cell therapy in thymic tumors.

c. Personalized Treatment Plans:

- Genomic and proteomic data guide the development of personalized treatment plans tailored to the unique molecular profiles of individual patients.

6. Genomic and Proteomic Technologies:

Advancements in genomic and proteomic technologies have accelerated research in thymic tumorigenesis:

a. Next-Generation Sequencing (NGS):

- NGS enables comprehensive genomic profiling, allowing for the detection of mutations, copy number alterations, and fusion genes.

b. Mass Spectrometry:

- Mass spectrometry-based proteomics offers high-throughput protein identification and quantification, facilitating biomarker discovery.

c. Liquid Biopsies:

- Liquid biopsies analyze circulating tumor DNA and proteins, providing non-invasive methods for monitoring disease progression and treatment response.

d. Single-Cell Analysis:

- Single-cell genomic and proteomic techniques allow for the characterization of individual tumor cells, revealing intratumoral heterogeneity.

7. Insights Gained from Genomic and Proteomic Research:

Genomic and proteomic research has yielded critical insights into thymic tumorigenesis:

a. Clonal Evolution:

- Understanding clonal evolution within thymic tumors has shed light on tumor progression and the emergence of treatment resistance.

b. Treatment Resistance Mechanisms:

- Genomic and proteomic studies have elucidated mechanisms of treatment resistance, guiding the development of strategies to overcome resistance.

c. Prognostic Markers:

- Identification of prognostic markers aids in stratifying patients based on their risk profile and guiding treatment decisions.

d. Target Discovery:

- Genomic and proteomic research has uncovered novel

therapeutic targets for drug development.

8. Challenges and Considerations:

Genomic and proteomic research in thymic tumorigenesis encounters challenges:

a. Tumor Heterogeneity:

- Thymic tumors exhibit significant intratumoral heterogeneity, necessitating comprehensive profiling.

b. Rare Malignancy:

- The rarity of thymic tumors poses challenges in obtaining sufficient samples for genomic and proteomic analyses.

c. Data Integration:

- Integrating multi-omics data (genomics, transcriptomics, proteomics) is complex but essential for a comprehensive understanding of tumor biology.

d. Clinical Translation:

- Translating genomic and proteomic findings into clinical practice requires rigorous validation and adaptation of treatment strategies.

9. Future Directions:

The future of genomic and proteomic research in thymic tumorigenesis holds promise:

a. Functional Characterization:

- Further elucidating the functional significance of genomic and proteomic alterations will provide deeper insights into disease mechanisms.

b. Multi-Omics Integration:

- Integration of genomics, transcriptomics, and proteomics data will enable a holistic understanding of thymic tumor biology.

c. Liquid Biopsy Advancements:

- Liquid biopsy technologies are expected to advance, offering non-invasive monitoring and early detection methods.

d. Clinical Trials:

- Clinical trials based on genomic and proteomic data will continue to evaluate novel therapies for thymic tumors.

10. Conclusion:

Genomic and proteomic research has been instrumental in unraveling the complexities of thymic tumorigenesis. It has identified key genetic alterations, characterized molecular subtypes, and informed the development of precision medicine approaches. As technology and techniques evolve, genomic and proteomic research will remain essential in improving the diagnosis, treatment, and outcomes of individuals with thymic tumors, offering hope for more effective therapies and enhanced quality of life.

11.4 Tumor Microenvironment Studies in Thymic Tumorigenesis

The tumor microenvironment (TME) is a dynamic and complex ecosystem surrounding cancer cells, playing a pivotal role in the development and progression of thymic tumors. Investigating the TME has provided crucial insights into the biology of these malignancies and opened new avenues for therapeutic interventions. In this section, we explore the significance of studying the TME in thymic tumorigenesis and its potential implications for treatment strategies.

1. Tumor Microenvironment:

The TME consists of a diverse array of cell types, including immune cells, fibroblasts, endothelial cells, and extracellular matrix components, all of which interact with cancer cells. Understanding these interactions is essential for comprehending cancer biology and designing effective therapies.

2. Cellular Components of the TME:

The TME in thymic tumors encompasses various cell types:

a. Immune Cells:

- Lymphocytes, macrophages, dendritic cells, and other immune cells infiltrate the TME, influencing tumor progression and immune responses.

b. Fibroblasts:

- Cancer-associated fibroblasts (CAFs) play a role in extracellular matrix remodeling and can contribute to tumor growth and invasion.

c. Endothelial Cells:

- Blood vessel formation within the TME is driven by endothelial cells, affecting tumor vascularization and nutrient supply.

d. Extracellular Matrix (ECM):

- The ECM provides structural support and signaling cues that can promote tumor cell survival and migration.

e. Secreted Factors:

- Soluble factors like cytokines, growth factors, and chemokines are produced within the TME, modulating tumor behavior.

3. Immunological Aspects of the TME:

The TME's immunological features have significant implications for thymic tumorigenesis:

a. Immune Infiltration:

- Characterizing the immune cell composition within thymic tumors can inform prognosis and treatment response.

b. Immune Suppression:

- Immunosuppressive mechanisms within the TME can hinder the body's ability to mount an effective antitumor immune response.

c. Immune Checkpoints:

- Immune checkpoint molecules, such as PD-1/PD-L1 and CTLA-4, are expressed within the TME and can be targeted with immunotherapy.

4. Stromal Components and Fibrosis:

The stromal components of the TME, including fibroblasts and the ECM, can contribute to thymic tumorigenesis:

a. Fibroblast Activation:

- CAFs can become activated and promote tumor growth, invasion, and drug resistance.

b. ECM Remodeling:

- Changes in the ECM can create a favorable environment for tumor cells, facilitating their survival and proliferation.

5. Angiogenesis and Vascularization:

The TME's influence on angiogenesis and vascularization is crucial in thymic tumorigenesis:

a. Tumor Angiogenesis:

- The formation of new blood vessels within the TME can supply nutrients and oxygen to tumor cells.

b. Vascular Permeability:

- Aberrant vascular permeability within the TME can lead to edema and affect drug delivery.

6. Hypoxia and Metabolic Adaptation:

The TME's influence on oxygen levels and metabolism has implications for tumor growth and treatment resistance:

a. Hypoxic Regions:

- Hypoxic areas within the TME can promote tumor cell survival and resistance to therapy.

b. Metabolic Reprogramming:

- Tumor cells may adapt to nutrient-deprived conditions through metabolic reprogramming.

7. Tumor-Associated Macrophages (TAMs):

TAMs are a key component of the TME with a dual role in thymic tumorigenesis:

a. Pro-Inflammatory M1 Macrophages:

- M1 macrophages can promote antitumor immune responses.

b. Anti-Inflammatory M2 Macrophages:

- M2 macrophages may have immunosuppressive properties that support tumor growth.

8. TME-Driven Immune Evasion Mechanisms:

The TME can employ various mechanisms to evade immune surveillance:

a. Immune Checkpoint Activation:

- Immune checkpoint molecules in the TME, such as PD-L1, can inhibit T-cell responses.

b. Regulatory T Cells (Tregs):

- Tregs within the TME can suppress antitumor immune responses.

c. Myeloid-Derived Suppressor Cells (MDSCs):

- MDSCs can inhibit immune cell functions and promote an immunosuppressive TME.

9. Biomarker Discovery:

Studying the TME offers opportunities for biomarker discovery:

a. Prognostic Biomarkers:

- TME-associated biomarkers can aid in predicting patient prognosis and treatment response.

b. Predictive Biomarkers:

- Biomarkers within the TME may predict how patients will respond to specific therapies, such as immunotherapy.

c. Therapeutic Targets:

- Components of the TME can serve as potential therapeutic targets, including immune checkpoints and stromal elements.

10. Immunotherapy Approaches:

The TME's role in immune evasion has prompted the development of immunotherapy strategies:

a. Immune Checkpoint Inhibitors:

- Targeting immune checkpoint molecules within the TME has shown promise in thymic tumors.

b. CAR T-Cell Therapy:

- Chimeric antigen receptor (CAR) T-cell therapy can be designed to target specific antigens present in the TME.

c. Cytokine Therapy:

- Enhancing cytokine signaling within the TME can bolster antitumor immune responses.

11. Therapeutic Modulation of the TME:

Therapeutic strategies can aim to modify the TME to enhance treatment efficacy:

a. Targeting Fibroblasts:

- Strategies to target CAFs or disrupt fibrosis may improve drug delivery and hinder tumor growth.

b. Normalizing Vasculature:

- Normalizing tumor vasculature can improve oxygen and drug delivery.

c. Combating Hypoxia:

- Strategies to alleviate hypoxia within the TME may sensitize tumors to radiation and chemotherapy.

12. Challenges and Considerations:

Studying the TME in thymic tumorigenesis presents several challenges:

a. Spatial Heterogeneity:

- The TME's composition can vary spatially within a tumor, requiring comprehensive analysis.

b. Dynamic Changes:

- The TME can evolve over time in response to therapy, impacting treatment efficacy.

c. Translational Barriers:

- Translating TME-focused research into clinical practice poses challenges in terms of therapeutic interventions.

13. Future Directions:

The future of TME studies in thymic tumorigenesis holds promise:

a. Single-Cell Analysis:

- Advancements in single-cell analysis techniques will provide insights into the heterogeneity of TME cell populations.

b. Combination Therapies:

- Combining therapies that target both tumor cells and

the TME may enhance treatment responses.

c. Personalized Approaches:

- Tailoring therapies based on TME characteristics may optimize treatment outcomes.

14. Conclusion:

The TME is a dynamic and multifaceted component of thymic tumorigenesis that influences tumor behavior, immune responses, and treatment outcomes. Understanding the intricacies of the TME offers opportunities for developing targeted therapies and personalized treatment approaches. As research in this field advances, we can anticipate improved strategies for managing thymic tumors and enhancing patient quality of life.

11.5 Therapeutic Development from Basic Research in Thymic Tumorigenesis

Thymic tumors, encompassing thymomas and thymic carcinomas, are rare malignancies that have historically posed significant challenges in terms of treatment. However, recent advancements in basic research have opened new horizons for therapeutic development. In this section, we explore how insights from basic research have translated into promising therapeutic strategies for thymic tumors, offering hope to patients with these uncommon cancers.

1. The Need for Therapeutic Advancements in Thymic Tumors

Thymic tumors are characterized by their rarity and diverse clinical behaviors. Conventional treatment options, including surgery, chemotherapy, and radiation therapy, have limitations in terms of efficacy and long-term outcomes. The development of targeted therapies and immunotherapies has been hampered by the lack of understanding of the molecular underpinnings of thymic tumorigenesis. However, recent advances in basic research have shed light on critical pathways and potential therapeutic targets, driving the development of innovative treatment approaches.

2. Insights from Genomic Studies: Precision Medicine in Thymic Tumors

Genomic research has revealed a wealth of information about the genetic alterations driving thymic tumors. Some key findings and their implications for therapeutic development include:

a. Mutations in Key Genes:

- Mutations in genes such as TP53, KIT, EGFR, and HRAS have been identified in thymic tumors. These mutations serve as potential targets for precision medicine approaches.

b. Molecular Subtypes:

- Molecular subtypes of thymic tumors, including type A, AB, B1, B2, B3 thymomas, and thymic carcinomas, have distinct genomic profiles. Tailoring therapies based on these subtypes may improve treatment outcomes.

c. Targeted Therapies:

- Genomic data have led to the development of targeted therapies that specifically inhibit aberrant signaling pathways. For instance, EGFR inhibitors and mTOR inhibitors are being investigated in clinical trials for thymic tumors with EGFR mutations.

d. Immunotherapy Targets:

- Genomic studies have identified potential immunotherapy targets, including immune checkpoint molecules such as PD-1 and PD-L1. Immune checkpoint inhibitors have shown promise in clinical trials for thymic tumors.

3. Immunotherapy Advancements: Harnessing the Immune System

Immunotherapy has emerged as a groundbreaking approach in the treatment of various cancers, including thymic tumors. Basic research has contributed to our understanding of immunological aspects, enabling the development of immunotherapeutic strategies:

a. Immune Checkpoint Inhibitors:

- Basic research on immune checkpoint molecules, such as PD-1/PD-L1 and CTLA-4, has paved the way for clinical trials involving checkpoint inhibitors in thymic tumors. Early results have shown encouraging responses in some patients.

b. CAR T-Cell Therapy:

- CAR T-cell therapy involves genetically engineering patients' T cells to target specific antigens expressed on tumor cells. Basic research on antigen expression in thymic tumors has laid the groundwork for the development of CAR T-cell therapies.

c. Combination Therapies:

- Basic research has highlighted the potential benefits of combining immunotherapies with other treatments, such as targeted therapies or radiation therapy, to enhance antitumor immune responses.

4. Targeting the Tumor Microenvironment: Insights from

TME Studies

The tumor microenvironment (TME) plays a crucial role in tumor development and treatment response. Basic research on the TME of thymic tumors has led to novel therapeutic strategies:

a. Targeting Immune Suppression:

- Research on immune-suppressive mechanisms within the TME, such as regulatory T cells (Tregs) and myeloid-derived suppressor cells (MDSCs), has prompted the investigation of therapies that counteract immune suppression.

b. Stromal Component Modulation:

- Basic research on cancer-associated fibroblasts (CAFs) and extracellular matrix (ECM) remodeling within the TME has led to strategies aimed at disrupting CAF-ECM interactions to hinder tumor growth and metastasis.

c. Normalizing Vasculature:

- Insights into tumor angiogenesis have guided the development of therapies aimed at normalizing tumor vasculature, improving drug delivery and oxygenation.

5. Biomarker Discovery and Personalized Medicine: Translating Research to Patient Care

Basic research has contributed to the identification of potential biomarkers for thymic tumors, aiding in personalized treatment approaches:

a. Prognostic Biomarkers:

- Biomarkers associated with patient prognosis have the potential to guide treatment decisions and surveillance strategies.

b. Predictive Biomarkers:

- Biomarkers predictive of treatment response can help tailor therapies to individual patients, optimizing outcomes and minimizing adverse effects.

c. Patient Stratification:

- Molecular profiling of tumors allows for patient stratification based on genomic profiles, ensuring that treatments are matched to the specific characteristics of each tumor.

6. Preclinical Models: Bridging the Gap from Bench to Bedside

Basic research has contributed to the development of preclinical models that mimic thymic tumors, facilitating the testing of potential therapies:

a. Patient-Derived Xenografts (PDX):

- PDX models involve transplanting patient tumor tissue into mice, allowing researchers to evaluate the efficacy of treatments in a context that closely resembles human tumors.

b. Genetically Engineered Mouse Models (GEMMs):

- GEMMs are engineered to develop thymic tumors, providing insights into disease mechanisms and enabling the preclinical evaluation of novel therapies.

7. Challenges and Considerations: Overcoming Hurdles in Therapeutic Development

While basic research has brought about significant advancements in thymic tumor therapeutics, several challenges persist:

a. Tumor Heterogeneity:

- Thymic tumors exhibit considerable heterogeneity, making it essential to develop therapies that account for this diversity.

b. Resistance Mechanisms:

- Tumors can develop resistance to targeted therapies and immunotherapies over time, necessitating ongoing research to overcome resistance mechanisms.

c. Clinical Translation:

- Translating promising findings from basic research into clinically effective therapies requires rigorous testing in human trials.

d. Rare Disease Status:

- The rarity of thymic tumors can pose challenges in conducting large-scale clinical trials and obtaining sufficient patient cohorts for research.

8. Future Directions: Advancing Therapeutic Development

The future of therapeutic development in thymic tumors holds several promising directions:

a. Combination Therapies:

- Investigating the synergy between different treatment modalities, such as targeted therapies, immunotherapies, and radiation therapy, may lead to more effective combination regimens.

b. Liquid Biopsies:

- Advancements in liquid biopsy techniques can provide

non-invasive monitoring of disease progression and treatment response, guiding real-time therapeutic adjustments.

c. Personalized Medicine:

- Further refinements in molecular profiling and biomarker discovery will enable increasingly personalized treatment approaches.

d. Clinical Trials:

- Expanding the number of clinical trials for thymic tumors, particularly those testing novel therapies, will be crucial for advancing treatment options.

9. Conclusion: Bridging the Gap Between Research and Clinical Impact

Basic research has significantly advanced our understanding of thymic tumorigenesis and provided a foundation for innovative therapeutic strategies. The combination of precision medicine, immunotherapy, and insights from the tumor microenvironment has opened new avenues for treating thymic tumors, offering hope to patients with these rare malignancies. As research continues to evolve, we anticipate continued improvements in thymic tumor therapeutics, ultimately leading to better outcomes and enhanced quality of life for affected individuals.

11.6 Collaborative Efforts in Thymic Tumor Research

Collaboration is a cornerstone of progress in medical research, and it holds particular significance in the context of rare and complex diseases such as thymic tumors. In this section, we delve into the importance of collaborative efforts in thymic tumor research, exploring how multidisciplinary collaborations, international consortia, and patient advocacy groups have played pivotal roles in advancing our understanding of these rare malignancies and improving patient care.

1. The Rarity and Complexity of Thymic Tumors

Thymic tumors are a group of rare malignancies that originate in the thymus gland, an essential component of the immune system. Due to their rarity and diverse clinical behaviors, thymic tumors have presented unique challenges to researchers and clinicians. However, collaborative efforts have emerged as a powerful force driving progress in thymic tumor research.

2. Multidisciplinary Collaboration: A Holistic Approach

Multidisciplinary collaboration involves experts from various fields coming together to address complex medical challenges comprehensively. In thymic tumor research, this approach has proven to be invaluable:

a. Clinical Oncology Teams:

- Oncologists, surgeons, and radiation oncologists collaborate to provide the best treatment options for patients. Multidisciplinary tumor boards ensure that treatment plans are tailored to individual cases.

b. Pathologists and Histologists:

- Pathologists play a pivotal role in diagnosing thymic tumors and assessing their histological subtypes. Collaboration with clinicians is essential for accurate diagnosis and treatment decisions.

c. Radiologists:

- Radiologists use advanced imaging techniques to

assist in staging and monitoring thymic tumors. Collaboration with oncologists is crucial for interpreting imaging results.

d. Basic and Translational Researchers:

- Collaboration between basic scientists and clinicians fosters the translation of laboratory discoveries into clinical applications. Basic research informs clinical trials and therapeutic development.

3. International Consortia: Uniting Global Efforts

The rarity of thymic tumors has prompted the formation of international consortia, bringing together researchers, clinicians, and institutions from around the world. These consortia have several key objectives:

a. Data Sharing:

- International consortia facilitate the sharing of patient data, tissue samples, and research findings. This global collaboration expands the pool of data available for analysis, enabling more comprehensive research.

b. Harmonization of Protocols:

- Standardized protocols for diagnosis, treatment, and research ensure consistency and comparability across institutions. This harmonization is particularly crucial for rare diseases like thymic tumors.

c. Large-Scale Studies:

- Consortia can pool resources to conduct large-scale studies, allowing for more robust statistical analyses and a deeper understanding of disease characteristics.

d. Clinical Trials:

- International collaborations enable the design and execution of clinical trials with larger patient cohorts, increasing the statistical power to detect treatment effects.

4. Patient Advocacy Groups: A Voice for Patients

Patient advocacy groups are instrumental in thymic tumor research, serving as advocates for patients, raising awareness, and supporting research initiatives:

a. Raising Awareness:

- Patient advocacy groups play a vital role in raising awareness about thymic tumors among the public and medical community. Increased awareness can lead to earlier diagnosis and improved access to specialized care.

b. Fundraising:

- Advocacy groups often engage in fundraising activities to support research efforts. These funds can be directed toward basic research, clinical trials, and patient support services.

c. Patient Empowerment:

- Patient advocacy groups empower individuals affected by thymic tumors by providing information, resources, and a sense of community. Empowered patients can actively participate in their healthcare decisions.

d. Collaboration with Researchers:

- Advocacy groups collaborate with researchers to identify research priorities, facilitate patient enrollment in clinical trials, and provide valuable patient perspectives to inform research directions.

5. Advances in Genomic Research: A Collaborative Frontier

Genomic research in thymic tumors has benefited greatly from collaborative efforts:

a. Genomic Data Sharing:

- International initiatives, such as The Cancer Genome Atlas (TCGA), have provided platforms for sharing genomic data from thymic tumors. This data sharing accelerates research by providing access to large-scale genomic information.

b. Collaborative Sequencing Projects:

- Researchers from multiple institutions collaborate on sequencing projects to identify genetic mutations and variations specific to thymic tumors. These efforts have revealed potential therapeutic targets.

c. Genomic Consortia:

- Genomic consortia, consisting of researchers with expertise in genomics and cancer biology, focus on deciphering the genomic landscape of thymic tumors. These consortia facilitate cross-disciplinary collaboration.

d. Biomarker Discovery:

- Collaboration between genomics experts and clinicians has led to the discovery of biomarkers that can aid in diagnosis, prognosis, and treatment decisions.

6. Challenges and Ethical Considerations:

Despite the many benefits of collaboration, challenges and ethical considerations must be addressed:

a. Data Privacy:

- Protecting patient privacy while sharing sensitive medical data is a critical concern. International consortia must adhere to stringent data protection regulations.

b. Research Disparities:

- Collaborations should strive to include researchers from diverse geographic regions to prevent disparities in research contributions and access to benefits.

c. Resource Allocation:

- The allocation of resources, including funding and research support, can be a source of contention in collaborative efforts. Transparent resource allocation processes are essential.

d. Ethical Research Conduct:

- Ethical considerations, such as informed consent and adherence to research ethics guidelines, must be at the forefront of collaborative research.

7. Future Directions: Expanding Collaborative Networks

The future of collaborative efforts in thymic tumor research holds great promise:

a. Integration of Multi-Omics Data:

- Collaborative research will integrate genomics, transcriptomics, proteomics, and other omics data to create a holistic understanding of thymic tumors.

b. Global Clinical Trials:

- International consortia will continue to drive the

design and execution of global clinical trials, evaluating novel therapies for thymic tumors.

c. Patient-Centered Research:

- Collaboration with patient advocacy groups will increasingly incorporate patient perspectives into research, ensuring that studies align with patient needs and priorities.

d. Targeted Therapies:

- Genomic insights will lead to the development of targeted therapies tailored to specific molecular subtypes of thymic tumors.

e. Personalized Medicine:

- Collaborative research will pave the way for personalized treatment approaches, optimizing therapeutic efficacy and minimizing side effects.

8. Conclusion: The Power of Collaboration in Thymic Tumor Research

Collaboration is at the heart of progress in thymic tumor research. Multidisciplinary teams, international consortia, and patient advocacy groups have collectively advanced our understanding of these rare malignancies and accelerated the development of innovative therapies. As we look to the future, continued collaboration holds the key to improving outcomes and enhancing the quality of life for individuals affected by thymic tumors. By fostering partnerships and leveraging collective expertise, we can overcome the challenges posed by these rare diseases and bring hope to patients and their families.

CHAPTER 12: GLOBAL PERSPECTIVES AND FUTURE DIRECTIONS

12.1 International Trends in Thymic Tumor Management

Thymic tumors, encompassing thymomas and thymic carcinomas, are rare malignancies that require a multidisciplinary approach to treatment. As our understanding of these tumors evolves, international trends in their management have emerged. In this section, we explore the latest international trends in the diagnosis, treatment, and research of thymic tumors, highlighting advances in precision medicine, immunotherapy, and collaborative efforts.

1. The Global Perspective on Thymic Tumor Management

Thymic tumors, while rare, pose unique challenges to clinicians and researchers worldwide. Their clinical behavior can range from indolent to aggressive, necessitating tailored approaches to management. International collaboration and the sharing of knowledge have become increasingly essential in addressing these challenges.

2. Multidisciplinary Care: A Universal Approach

Internationally, multidisciplinary care has become the gold standard in managing thymic tumors. This approach involves a collaborative team of healthcare professionals, including oncologists, surgeons, radiologists, pathologists, and specialized nurses. The benefits of multidisciplinary care are consistent across borders:

a. Comprehensive Evaluation:

- Multidisciplinary teams assess each patient's case comprehensively, considering factors such as tumor size, histological subtype, stage, and individual patient characteristics.

b. Tailored Treatment Plans:

- Treatment recommendations are customized based on a patient's specific tumor characteristics and overall health. This approach optimizes treatment outcomes.

c. Shared Decision-Making:

- Patients are actively involved in treatment decisions, with healthcare providers explaining the risks, benefits, and alternatives for each therapeutic option.

d. Ongoing Monitoring:

- Multidisciplinary teams ensure that patients receive continuous monitoring and follow-up care, even after treatment completion.

3. Advances in Molecular Profiling: Precision Medicine in Thymic Tumors

One of the most significant international trends in thymic tumor management is the incorporation of precision medicine. Molecular profiling and targeted therapies have gained prominence:

a. Genomic Analysis:

- Internationally, genomic analysis of thymic tumors has become routine practice. Tumor tissue is sequenced to identify genetic mutations, alterations, and molecular subtypes.

b. Targeted Therapies:

- Based on genomic findings, targeted therapies are increasingly used in thymic tumor management. For example, EGFR inhibitors, mTOR inhibitors, and immunotherapies are explored for specific molecular subgroups.

c. Personalized Treatment Plans:

- Physicians across borders are tailoring treatment plans to each patient's genomic profile. This personalized approach enhances treatment efficacy while minimizing side effects.

d. Emerging Biomarkers:

- International research efforts continue to identify novel biomarkers associated with thymic tumors, aiding in prognosis and treatment selection.

4. Immunotherapy Revolution: Harnessing the Immune System

Immunotherapy has revolutionized cancer treatment globally, and thymic tumors are no exception. International trends in thymic tumor management include the integration of immunotherapies:

a. Immune Checkpoint Inhibitors:

- Immune checkpoint inhibitors, such as PD-1/PD-L1 and CTLA-4 inhibitors, have shown promising results in thymic tumor patients internationally. These therapies unleash the immune system against cancer cells.

b. CAR T-Cell Therapy:

- CAR T-cell therapy, designed to target specific antigens on tumor cells, is being explored internationally as a potential treatment modality for thymic tumors.

c. Combination Therapies:

- Internationally, clinical trials are investigating combinations of immunotherapies with other treatments, such as chemotherapy, radiation therapy, or targeted therapies, to enhance antitumor immune responses.

d. Real-World Data:

- International collaborative efforts are collecting real-world data on immunotherapy outcomes in thymic tumor patients to refine treatment guidelines and optimize patient care.

5. Collaborative Research Consortia: Global Insights

International collaboration in research consortia is pivotal to advancing thymic tumor management. Key aspects of these consortia include:

a. Data Sharing:

- Researchers worldwide are sharing patient data, tissue samples, and research findings. This global cooperation expands the dataset available for analysis.

b. Large-Scale Studies:

- International consortia can pool resources to conduct large-scale studies, allowing for more robust statistical analyses and a deeper understanding of disease characteristics.

c. Harmonization of Protocols:

- Standardized protocols for diagnosis, treatment, and research ensure consistency and comparability across institutions and countries.

d. Clinical Trials:

- Collaborative international trials have the advantage of larger patient cohorts, increasing the statistical power to detect treatment effects.

6. Patient Advocacy on a Global Scale

Patient advocacy groups have a global presence in the landscape of thymic tumor management:

a. Raising Global Awareness:

- These groups work collectively to raise awareness about thymic tumors on a global scale. Increased awareness can lead to earlier diagnosis and improved access to specialized care.

b. Global Fundraising:

- Advocacy groups engage in fundraising efforts with an international reach. These funds support research, patient support services, and awareness campaigns.

c. International Support:

- Patient advocacy groups collaborate internationally to share resources, provide patient support, and advocate for research funding.

d. Global Research Engagement:

- These groups play a vital role in connecting patients with international research efforts, facilitating patient participation in clinical trials and research studies.

7. Challenges and Opportunities in International Trends

While international collaboration in thymic tumor management is promising, challenges persist:

a. Resource Disparities:

- Disparities in healthcare infrastructure and resources across countries can impact patient outcomes and access to cutting-edge treatments.

b. Regulatory Variations:

- Differences in regulatory processes and approval timelines for new therapies can create delays in international treatment options.

c. Data Privacy:

- Ensuring the privacy and security of patient data while sharing it across borders is a complex ethical and legal challenge.

d. Access to Care:

- Ensuring that patients worldwide have equitable access to the latest advancements in thymic tumor management remains a goal for international collaboration.

8. Future Directions: A Global Approach to Thymic Tumor Management

The future of thymic tumor management is undeniably global:

a. Targeted Therapies:

- International research will continue to identify and refine targeted therapies tailored to specific molecular subtypes of thymic tumors.

b. Immunotherapy Advancements:

- Collaborative international efforts will drive the development of novel immunotherapies and combination treatments for thymic tumors.

c. Real-World Evidence:

- The accumulation of real-world data from diverse patient populations will inform treatment guidelines and strategies.

d. Rare Disease Networks:

- International networks and consortia focused on rare diseases, including thymic tumors, will grow in influence, advancing research and patient care.

9. Conclusion: A Unified Effort for Thymic Tumor Patients

International trends in thymic tumor management reflect a collective effort to improve outcomes for patients facing these rare malignancies. By sharing knowledge, resources, and expertise across borders, clinicians, researchers, and patient advocates are working together to transform thymic tumor management on a global scale. As these international collaborations continue to evolve, we can anticipate better treatments, improved access to care, and a brighter future for individuals affected by thymic tumors worldwide.

12.2 Disparities in Access to Care for Thymic Tumor Patients

Thymic tumors, a group of rare malignancies arising from the thymus gland, present unique challenges in terms of diagnosis and treatment. While significant progress has been made in understanding and managing these tumors, disparities in access to care persist, affecting patients' outcomes and quality of life. This section delves into the disparities that thymic tumor patients face worldwide, exploring the reasons behind these inequalities and proposing strategies to address them.

1. The Global Impact of Disparities

Disparities in healthcare access and outcomes are a global concern that affects a wide range of diseases, including rare malignancies like thymic tumors. These disparities are rooted in various factors, from socioeconomic status and geography to healthcare infrastructure and policy.

2. Socioeconomic Disparities: A Barrier to Equitable Care

Socioeconomic disparities play a significant role in access to care for thymic tumor patients. Key points to consider include:

a. Financial Barriers:

- Thymic tumor treatment can be expensive, involving surgery, radiation therapy, chemotherapy, targeted therapies, and immunotherapies. Patients with limited financial resources may struggle to access and afford these treatments.

b. Health Insurance:

- Lack of health insurance coverage or underinsurance can lead to delayed or inadequate care for thymic tumor patients. High out-of-pocket costs can deter individuals from seeking medical attention.

c. Geographic Location:

- Patients in rural or underserved areas may face challenges in accessing specialized healthcare facilities and expertise, including thymic tumor specialists.

d. Educational Disparities:

- Limited health literacy and awareness about thymic tumors can hinder early diagnosis and timely treatment initiation.

3. Healthcare Infrastructure and Expertise: A Global Divide

Access to specialized healthcare infrastructure and expertise varies significantly across countries and regions:

a. Concentration of Expertise:

- Thymic tumor expertise is often concentrated in specialized cancer centers or academic medical institutions, which may not be accessible to all patients, especially those in remote areas.

b. Availability of Treatment Modalities:

- Access to state-of-the-art treatments, including targeted therapies and immunotherapies, can be limited in certain healthcare systems.

c. Diagnostic Facilities:

- Timely and accurate diagnosis of thymic tumors requires access to advanced diagnostic facilities, such as PET-CT scanners and molecular profiling services.

d. Limited Clinical Trials:

- Participation in clinical trials, which can offer cutting-edge treatments, is often limited to patients in specific regions or countries.

4. Racial and Ethnic Disparities: A Complex Issue

Racial and ethnic disparities in healthcare access and outcomes are multifaceted and influenced by various factors, including:

a. Cultural Factors:

- Language barriers and cultural differences can affect communication with healthcare providers and adherence to treatment plans.

b. Implicit Bias:

- Implicit biases among healthcare professionals can lead to differences in the care provided to patients from diverse racial and ethnic backgrounds.

c. Socioeconomic Factors:

- Racial and ethnic minorities may face higher rates of poverty and limited access to healthcare insurance, exacerbating disparities.

d. Health System Inequities:

- Structural inequities within healthcare systems can result in unequal access to quality care.

5. Gender Disparities: An Underexplored Aspect

Gender disparities in thymic tumor care are an underexplored aspect of healthcare disparities. While thymic tumors are rare, they can affect individuals of all genders. Factors to consider include:

a. Treatment Decisions:

- Gender bias may influence treatment decisions, affecting the choice of surgical approaches, access to clinical trials, and follow-up care.

b. Survivorship and Quality of Life:

- Gender-specific survivorship and quality-of-life issues may not be adequately addressed in thymic tumor care.

c. Representation in Research:

- Clinical trials and research studies may not always include diverse gender populations, limiting our understanding of gender-specific aspects of thymic tumors.

6. Strategies to Address Disparities

Addressing disparities in access to care for thymic tumor patients requires a multi-pronged approach at the local, national, and global levels:

a. Education and Awareness:

- Public health campaigns and educational initiatives can increase awareness about thymic tumors, leading to earlier diagnosis and treatment.

b. Supportive Services:

- Providing social support, transportation assistance, and financial counseling can alleviate some of the socioeconomic barriers to care.

c. Telehealth and Telemedicine:

- Expanding telehealth services can help patients in remote areas access expert consultations and follow-up care.

d. Healthcare Policy:

- Governments and healthcare policymakers can implement policies to reduce financial barriers, expand insurance coverage, and incentivize the establishment of specialized thymic tumor centers.

e. Cultural Competence Training:

- Healthcare providers should receive cultural competence training to better serve patients from diverse racial, ethnic, and cultural backgrounds.

f. Research Equity:

- Ensuring equitable inclusion of diverse populations in clinical trials and research studies is essential for understanding and addressing disparities.

g. Patient Advocacy:

- Patient advocacy groups can play a crucial role in raising awareness about disparities and advocating for policy changes and equitable access to care.

7. International Collaboration: A Global Effort

Given that thymic tumors are rare, international collaboration is essential in addressing disparities:

a. Knowledge Sharing:

- Collaborative networks can facilitate the sharing of best practices, treatment protocols, and research findings across borders.

b. Telemedicine Solutions:

- Telemedicine initiatives can connect patients with expert clinicians and specialists worldwide, reducing geographic disparities.

c. Global Clinical Trials:

- International clinical trials can offer patients access to novel treatments and therapies, regardless of their location.

d. Advocacy on a Global Scale:

- International patient advocacy groups can raise awareness about disparities and advocate for equitable care on a global scale.

8. Conclusion: Toward Equitable Care for Thymic Tumor Patients

Disparities in access to care for thymic tumor patients are a complex and multifaceted issue with global implications. While challenges persist, concerted efforts at the local, national, and international levels can help bridge these gaps. By addressing socioeconomic, racial, ethnic, and gender disparities and fostering collaboration among healthcare providers, researchers, policymakers, and patient advocates, we can strive for more equitable care and improved outcomes for individuals affected by thymic tumors worldwide.

12.3 Multinational Collaborations and Research Networks in Thymic Tumor Research

Thymic tumors, encompassing thymomas and thymic carcinomas, are rare and complex malignancies that require a global effort to advance our understanding and treatment options. Multinational collaborations and research networks have emerged as crucial components of this effort, allowing researchers, clinicians, and patient advocates from different countries to work together in addressing the challenges posed by these rare diseases. In this section, we explore the significance, achievements, and future potential of multinational collaborations and research networks in thymic tumor research.

1. The Global Challenge of Thymic Tumors

Thymic tumors are characterized by their rarity and heterogeneity, making research and treatment advancements particularly challenging. These malignancies affect individuals worldwide, and the complexity of their biology necessitates a unified global approach to improve patient outcomes.

2. The Significance of Multinational Collaborations

Multinational collaborations bring together experts and resources from various countries to tackle the multifaceted challenges posed by thymic tumors. The significance of such collaborations is evident in several key aspects:

a. Pooling of Expertise:

- Multinational collaborations allow the pooling of expertise from different regions, ensuring that a diverse range of perspectives and knowledge is applied to thymic tumor research.

b. Access to Diverse Patient Populations:

- Collaborations encompassing multiple countries provide access to diverse patient populations, which is essential for conducting meaningful clinical trials and research studies.

c. Resource Sharing:

- Collaboration facilitates the sharing of resources, including research funding, clinical data, tissue samples, and access to advanced technologies and equipment.

d. Accelerated Progress:

- Multinational collaborations accelerate progress by enabling larger-scale studies, more extensive data collection, and faster recruitment of patients for clinical trials.

e. International Consensus:

- Collaboration fosters international consensus on diagnostic criteria, treatment protocols, and research priorities, ensuring uniformity in thymic tumor management.

3. Achievements and Milestones

Multinational collaborations in thymic tumor research have already achieved significant milestones:

a. Standardized Diagnostic Criteria:

- Collaborative efforts have led to the development of standardized diagnostic criteria, enabling consistent and accurate diagnosis of thymic tumors across borders.

b. Collaborative Clinical Trials:

- Multinational clinical trials have been conducted to evaluate novel treatments and therapies for thymic tumors, offering patients access to cutting-edge interventions.

c. Genomic Profiling Initiatives:

- Research networks have undertaken genomic profiling initiatives, identifying key genetic alterations and molecular subtypes of thymic tumors.

d. Biomarker Discovery:

- Collaborative research has resulted in the discovery of biomarkers that aid in diagnosis, prognosis, and treatment selection for thymic tumors.

e. Global Patient Registries:

- International patient registries have been established to collect comprehensive data on thymic tumor patients, enabling more in-depth analyses and long-term follow-up.

4. International Research Networks: Leading the Way

Several international research networks have been at the forefront of thymic tumor research, driving progress and innovation:

a. ITMIG (International Thymic Malignancy Interest Group):

- ITMIG is a global organization dedicated to the study of thymic malignancies. It brings together experts from various disciplines, promoting research, collaboration, and education in the field.

b. IASLC (International Association for the Study of Lung Cancer):

- IASLC includes researchers and clinicians focused on lung cancer and thymic tumors. Their work contributes to a comprehensive understanding of thoracic malignancies.

c. Rare Cancer Network:

- The Rare Cancer Network is a global alliance of medical professionals and researchers dedicated to rare cancers, including thymic tumors. It facilitates collaborative research and clinical trials.

d. TETC (Thymic Epithelial Tumor Collaborative):

- TETC is a research consortium dedicated to advancing thymic tumor research. It emphasizes the importance of collaboration among clinicians, researchers, and patient advocates.

5. The Role of Patient Advocacy Groups

Patient advocacy groups have played a vital role in fostering multinational collaborations in thymic tumor research:

a. Global Awareness:

- These groups raise global awareness about thymic tumors, ensuring that patients worldwide have access to information and support.

b. Connection and Support:

- International patient advocacy networks connect individuals affected by thymic tumors, providing a sense of community and emotional support.

c. Research Advocacy:

- Patient advocates actively participate in collaborative research initiatives, sharing their insights and priorities with researchers and clinicians.

d. Fundraising:

- Advocacy groups engage in global fundraising efforts to support research, clinical trials, and patient support services.

6. Challenges and Future Directions

Despite the successes of multinational collaborations, challenges persist:

a. Resource Disparities:

- Resource disparities among countries can hinder equitable participation in collaborative research efforts.

b. Regulatory Hurdles:

- Differences in regulatory processes and approval

timelines for clinical trials can slow down international research initiatives.

c. Data Privacy:

- Protecting patient privacy while sharing medical data across borders remains a complex ethical and legal challenge.

d. Health Inequities:

- Addressing broader health inequities, such as access to basic healthcare services, is crucial for improving thymic tumor outcomes on a global scale.

e. Sustaining Collaboration:

- Sustaining long-term collaboration requires ongoing commitment and coordination among international partners.

7. The Future of Multinational Collaborations in Thymic Tumor Research

The future of multinational collaborations in thymic tumor research holds great promise:

a. Targeted Therapies:

- Collaborative efforts will continue to identify and refine targeted therapies tailored to specific molecular subtypes of thymic tumors.

b. Immunotherapy Advancements:

- International networks will drive the development of novel immunotherapies and combination treatments for thymic tumors.

c. Real-World Evidence:

- The accumulation of real-world data from diverse patient populations will inform treatment guidelines and strategies.

d. Global Networks:

- The expansion of international research networks will enhance knowledge exchange and collaborative research on thymic tumors.

e. Patient-Centered Research:

- Multinational collaborations will increasingly involve patients in research design, ensuring that studies address their needs and priorities.

8. Conclusion: A Global Front in Thymic Tumor Research

Multinational collaborations and research networks are at the forefront of advancing thymic tumor research and improving patient outcomes on a global scale. By fostering international cooperation, sharing knowledge and resources, and engaging with patient advocates, researchers and clinicians are paving the way for a brighter future for individuals affected by thymic tumors worldwide. The global community's commitment to addressing the challenges posed by these rare malignancies offers hope for more effective treatments and improved quality of life for thymic tumor patients across borders.

12.4 Emerging Therapeutic Strategies on the Horizon for Thymic Tumors

Thymic tumors, encompassing thymomas and thymic carcinomas, represent a rare and challenging group of malignancies. Recent advances in our understanding of the molecular and immunological underpinnings of these tumors have led to the development of innovative therapeutic strategies. In this section, we explore the emerging therapeutic approaches on the horizon for thymic tumors, shedding light on novel treatments, precision medicine, and immunotherapies that hold promise for improving patient outcomes.

1. The Evolving Landscape of Thymic Tumor Therapies

The treatment landscape for thymic tumors has undergone significant evolution in recent years. While surgery remains a cornerstone of treatment, emerging therapeutic strategies are reshaping the way we approach these rare malignancies. These emerging strategies are driven by advancements in our understanding of thymic tumor biology and the development of targeted therapies and immunotherapies.

2. Targeted Therapies: Precision Medicine in Thymic Tumors

Precision medicine, which tailors treatment to an individual's specific tumor characteristics, has gained momentum in thymic tumor management:

a. EGFR Inhibitors:

- Epidermal Growth Factor Receptor (EGFR) inhibitors, such as gefitinib and erlotinib, have shown promise in treating thymic tumors with EGFR mutations. These targeted therapies disrupt the signaling pathways that drive tumor growth.

b. mTOR Inhibitors:

- Mammalian Target of Rapamycin (mTOR) inhibitors, including everolimus, have demonstrated efficacy in controlling thymic tumor progression, especially in cases with mTOR pathway activation.

c. Immunotherapy Combinations:

- Combining targeted therapies with immunotherapies, such as checkpoint inhibitors, is an emerging strategy to enhance treatment responses by unleashing the immune system against the tumor.

d. Molecular Profiling:

- Advances in genomic profiling help identify actionable mutations and molecular subtypes, enabling personalized treatment plans for thymic tumor patients.

3. Immunotherapies: Unleashing the Immune System

Immunotherapies have transformed the treatment landscape for various cancers, including thymic tumors:

a. Immune Checkpoint Inhibitors:

- Checkpoint inhibitors targeting PD-1/PD-L1 and CTLA-4 have shown remarkable efficacy in a subset of thymic tumor patients, leading to durable responses and improved survival.

b. CAR T-Cell Therapy:

- Chimeric Antigen Receptor (CAR) T-cell therapy, although in its early stages for thymic tumors, holds potential for targeting specific antigens expressed on tumor cells.

c. Combination Strategies:

- Combining checkpoint inhibitors with other immunotherapies or targeted therapies is being explored to enhance antitumor immune responses.

d. Predictive Biomarkers:

- Research is ongoing to identify predictive biomarkers

that can help select thymic tumor patients most likely to benefit from immunotherapies.

4. Antibody-Drug Conjugates (ADCs): Precision Weapons

ADCs represent a promising class of therapies in which monoclonal antibodies are linked to cytotoxic drugs:

a. Antibody Selection:

- Identifying antibodies that target specific antigens on thymic tumor cells allows for selective drug delivery.

b. Reduced Toxicity:

- ADCs deliver the cytotoxic payload directly to tumor cells, minimizing damage to healthy tissues and reducing side effects.

c. Clinical Trials:

- Several ADCs are in early-phase clinical trials for thymic tumors, offering potential new treatment options.

5. Epigenetic Modulators: Controlling Gene Expression

Epigenetic modifications, which regulate gene expression, are a focus of emerging research in thymic tumor therapy:

a. HDAC Inhibitors:

- Histone Deacetylase (HDAC) inhibitors can modify gene expression patterns and are being investigated as potential therapies for thymic tumors.

b. DNA Methyltransferase Inhibitors:

- Drugs that target DNA methylation processes are being explored to control tumor growth and alter gene expression in thymic tumors.

c. Combination Approaches:

- Combining epigenetic modulators with other therapies, such as immunotherapies or targeted agents, is a strategy to enhance treatment efficacy.

6. Tumor Microenvironment Modulation: Targeting the Niche

The tumor microenvironment plays a crucial role in cancer progression, and strategies to modify it are under investigation:

a. Angiogenesis Inhibitors:

- Targeting the formation of new blood vessels that supply tumors with nutrients is a potential avenue for thymic tumor therapy.

b. Stromal Disruption:

- Disrupting the supportive stroma around tumor cells may weaken their growth-promoting environment.

c. Immunomodulation:

- Modifying the tumor microenvironment to enhance immune cell infiltration and function is an emerging approach in thymic tumor research.

7. Clinical Trials and Collaborative Research

The development and evaluation of emerging therapeutic strategies for thymic tumors heavily rely on clinical trials and collaborative research efforts:

a. Global Clinical Trials:

- International collaboration in clinical trials allows patients worldwide to access novel treatments and therapies.

b. Rare Cancer Networks:

- Networks and consortia dedicated to rare cancers, including thymic tumors, facilitate collaborative research and data sharing.

c. Real-World Evidence:

- Collecting real-world data from diverse patient populations provides insights into treatment outcomes and guides clinical decision-making.

8. Challenges and Future Directions

While emerging therapeutic strategies hold promise, challenges must be addressed:

a. Biomarker Discovery:

- Identifying predictive biomarkers for treatment response remains a priority to optimize therapy selection.

b. Resistance Mechanisms:

- Understanding and overcoming resistance mechanisms to targeted therapies and immunotherapies is essential for long-term treatment success.

c. Access and Equity:

- Ensuring equitable access to emerging therapies for all thymic tumor patients, regardless of geographic location or socioeconomic status, is a pressing concern.

d. Combination Therapies:

- Determining the optimal combinations of therapies

and treatment sequences requires rigorous clinical investigation.

e. Survivorship Care:

- As treatments improve, survivorship care plans should address long-term quality of life and potential late effects.

9. Conclusion: A Promising Future

The landscape of thymic tumor therapy is evolving rapidly, with emerging therapeutic strategies offering hope for improved outcomes and quality of life for patients. As researchers and clinicians continue to unravel the molecular and immunological complexities of these rare malignancies, collaborative efforts, precision medicine approaches, and innovative therapies will play pivotal roles in shaping the future of thymic tumor management. With global cooperation, access to cutting-edge treatments, and a commitment to patient-centered care, we are on the brink of a promising era in thymic tumor therapy.

12.5 Patient Advocacy and Support Groups for Thymic Tumor Patients

Facing a thymic tumor diagnosis can be a daunting and isolating experience. Patient advocacy and support groups have emerged as vital resources for individuals and their families navigating the challenges of these rare malignancies. In this section, we explore the critical role played by patient advocacy organizations and support groups in providing information, emotional support, and empowerment to thymic tumor patients.

1. The Impact of Advocacy and Support

The journey of a thymic tumor patient is marked by

uncertainty, treatment decisions, and emotional upheaval. Patient advocacy organizations and support groups provide invaluable assistance in addressing these challenges. They offer a sense of community, access to expert information, and a platform for raising awareness about thymic tumors.

2. The Need for Patient Advocacy in Thymic Tumors

Thymic tumors are rare, and information about them can be limited. Patients and their families often struggle to find accurate and up-to-date resources. Advocacy organizations step in to bridge this gap:

a. Raising Awareness:

- Advocacy groups work tirelessly to raise awareness about thymic tumors among the public and healthcare professionals.

b. Information Dissemination:

- They provide reliable information about diagnosis, treatment options, clinical trials, and coping strategies to empower patients to make informed decisions.

c. Research Funding:

- Advocacy organizations often play a significant role in raising funds for thymic tumor research, driving advancements in treatment.

d. Policy Advocacy:

- They advocate for policies that improve patient access to quality care and promote research into rare cancers.

3. Patient Support Groups: A Lifeline for Emotional Well-being

Support groups offer a safe space for thymic tumor patients to share their experiences, fears, and triumphs:

a. Peer Support:

- Connecting with others who have walked a similar path can alleviate feelings of isolation and provide a sense of belonging.

b. Emotional Guidance:

- Support groups offer emotional guidance and coping strategies to help patients and families navigate the emotional toll of cancer.

c. Sharing Knowledge:

- Patients often share practical insights into managing side effects, finding healthcare providers, and accessing resources.

d. Family Support:

- These groups extend support to family members and caregivers who also grapple with the challenges of caregiving.

4. Prominent Thymic Tumor Advocacy Organizations

Several advocacy organizations have dedicated themselves to the cause of thymic tumor patients:

a. Thymic Tumor Foundation:

- The Thymic Tumor Foundation is a leading advocacy group focused on accelerating research, providing support, and raising awareness about thymic tumors.

b. Thymic Alliance:

- Thymic Alliance is committed to enhancing the lives of thymic tumor patients and their families through advocacy, education, and support.

c. Rare Cancer Network:

- The Rare Cancer Network is a global alliance of medical professionals and researchers dedicated to rare cancers, including thymic tumors.

5. Services Offered by Patient Advocacy Organizations

Patient advocacy organizations and support groups provide an array of services to address the unique needs of thymic tumor patients:

a. Information and Education:

- They offer educational resources, including brochures, webinars, and workshops, to help patients understand their condition and treatment options.

b. Peer-to-Peer Support:

- Through online forums, support groups, and helplines, patients can connect with others facing similar challenges.

c. Patient Navigation:

- Advocacy organizations often provide patient navigation services to help individuals find appropriate healthcare providers and treatment centers.

d. Financial Assistance:

- Some groups offer financial aid or guidance on managing medical expenses, which can be significant in cancer care.

e. Research Support:

- Advocacy organizations may fund research projects,

clinical trials, and registries specific to thymic tumors.

6. Engaging in Advocacy and Research

Patient advocacy groups actively participate in research initiatives and clinical trials:

a. Patient-Driven Research:

- Some organizations encourage patients to contribute to research by sharing their medical data and participating in studies.

b. Clinical Trial Access:

- Advocacy groups advocate for greater patient access to clinical trials, ensuring that emerging treatments are available to thymic tumor patients.

c. Research Collaboration:

- Collaborations between advocacy organizations and researchers promote the inclusion of patient perspectives in research design and priorities.

d. Raising Research Funds:

- Advocacy groups often organize fundraising events and campaigns to support thymic tumor research.

7. Challenges in Advocacy and Support

Despite their invaluable contributions, patient advocacy organizations face challenges:

a. Limited Resources:

- Many advocacy groups operate on limited budgets, restricting their ability to provide comprehensive services.

b. Rare Disease Status:

- The rarity of thymic tumors means that advocacy efforts may not receive the same attention and funding as more common cancers.

c. Geographic Barriers:

- Patients in remote or underserved areas may have limited access to advocacy services.

d. Access to Care:

- Advocacy organizations often grapple with addressing disparities in access to thymic tumor care, especially in regions with limited healthcare infrastructure.

8. Future Directions: A Unified Effort

The future of patient advocacy and support for thymic tumor patients holds great potential:

a. Global Collaboration:

- Advocacy organizations are increasingly collaborating on a global scale to pool resources, knowledge, and expertise.

b. Advocacy for Equity:

- Addressing disparities in access to care and advocating for equitable treatment options is a priority.

c. Expanded Research:

- Advocacy groups will continue to support and drive research efforts, contributing to a deeper understanding of thymic tumors.

d. Patient-Centered Care:

- The patient voice will continue to be central to advocacy and research, ensuring that patient needs and preferences guide decision-making.

9. Conclusion: A Beacon of Hope

Patient advocacy organizations and support groups are beacons of hope for thymic tumor patients and their families. In a journey marked by uncertainty, these organizations provide information, emotional support, and a sense of community. As the landscape of thymic tumor care continues to evolve, the vital role played by advocacy groups in driving research, raising awareness, and championing patient-centered care cannot be overstated. With their unwavering commitment, these organizations illuminate the path toward improved outcomes and a brighter future for thymic tumor patients.

12.6 A Vision for the Future: Towards Better Outcomes in Thymic Tumor Patients

The landscape of thymic tumor management is evolving rapidly, offering hope for improved outcomes, enhanced quality of life, and increased survival rates for patients facing these rare malignancies. In this final section, we envision a future where advancements in research, treatment modalities, and patient care converge to transform the journey of thymic tumor patients.

1. A Journey of Transformation

The vision for the future of thymic tumor patients is one of transformation—a journey from uncertainty and rarity to understanding, hope, and improved quality of life. This vision is driven by the collective efforts of researchers, clinicians, patient advocates, and the global healthcare community.

2. Early Detection and Screening

In the future, advancements in screening and early detection methods will play a pivotal role in improving thymic tumor outcomes:

a. Biomarker-Based Screening:

- Robust biomarkers will be identified, enabling non-invasive and accurate screening for individuals at risk.

b. Imaging Innovations:

- Cutting-edge imaging technologies will enhance the detection of small thymic tumors, allowing for earlier intervention.

c. Risk Assessment:

- Comprehensive risk assessment models will help identify individuals with genetic predispositions or environmental factors that increase their susceptibility to thymic tumors.

d. Personalized Screening Plans:

- Screening plans will be tailored to individual risk profiles, ensuring efficient and effective early detection strategies.

3. Precision Medicine: Tailored Treatments

The future of thymic tumor management will see the widespread implementation of precision medicine:

a. Targeted Therapies:

- A range of targeted therapies will be available, addressing specific genetic alterations and molecular subtypes of thymic tumors.

b. Immunotherapies:

- Immunotherapy approaches will be fine-tuned, with a focus on enhancing response rates and minimizing side effects.

c. Combination Treatments:

- Combinations of targeted therapies, immunotherapies, and traditional treatments will be optimized for individual patients, improving overall treatment outcomes.

d. Genomic Profiling:

- Routine genomic profiling will guide treatment decisions, ensuring that patients receive the therapies most likely to benefit them.

4. Patient-Centered Care

The vision for thymic tumor patient care is centered on the patient's experience and well-being:

a. Survivorship Programs:

- Comprehensive survivorship programs will address long-term quality of life, monitoring for late effects, and providing support for survivors.

b. Holistic Care:

- Holistic approaches to care will encompass not only physical health but also emotional, psychological, and social well-being.

c. Supportive Care Networks:

- Robust networks of patient advocates, support groups, and counselors will be available to provide guidance and support throughout the journey.

d. Inclusive Decision-Making:

- Patients will actively participate in shared decision-making, ensuring their values and preferences are integrated into their care plans.

5. Advancements in Research

The future of thymic tumor research will yield a deeper understanding of the disease and innovative treatments:

a. Personalized Clinical Trials:

- Clinical trials will be increasingly personalized, matching patients with trials based on their specific tumor characteristics.

b. Real-World Evidence:

- Real-world evidence from diverse patient populations will inform treatment guidelines and improve outcomes.

c. Molecular Insights:

- Ongoing research will uncover new molecular targets and pathways, expanding treatment options.

d. Collaborative Research Networks:

- International collaborations will continue to drive thymic tumor research, accelerating progress through shared knowledge and resources.

6. Global Access to Care

In the future, access to high-quality care for thymic tumor patients will be equitable, regardless of geographic location or socioeconomic status:

a. Telemedicine and Telehealth:

- Telehealth services will provide remote access to expert care, reducing geographic barriers.

b. Comprehensive Care Centers:

- Specialized thymic tumor care centers will be available in regions around the world, ensuring that patients receive the best possible treatment.

c. Health Equity Initiatives:

- Global health equity initiatives will focus on addressing disparities in access to care, diagnostics, and treatment.

d. Multinational Collaborations:

- Collaborations between countries and healthcare systems will facilitate the sharing of knowledge and resources, further improving access to care.

7. Data-Driven Decision-Making

The future of thymic tumor management will be characterized by data-driven decision-making at every stage:

a. Predictive Analytics:

- Advanced predictive analytics will help identify patients at risk for thymic tumors, allowing for early intervention.

b. Treatment Algorithms:

- Algorithms incorporating patient-specific data will guide treatment decisions, optimizing therapy selection.

c. Real-Time Monitoring:

- Real-time monitoring of patient data will enable rapid adjustments to treatment plans, improving outcomes.

d. Research Informatics:

- Big data and research informatics will facilitate the analysis of vast datasets, driving discoveries in thymic tumor research.

8. Education and Awareness

A future where thymic tumors are well-understood and recognized will rely on education and awareness efforts:

a. Medical Education:

- Thymic tumor education will be integrated into medical curricula, ensuring that healthcare professionals are well-prepared to diagnose and treat these rare malignancies.

b. Public Awareness Campaigns:

- Ongoing awareness campaigns will educate the public about thymic tumors, promoting early detection and timely treatment.

c. Patient Empowerment:

- Patient education will empower individuals to advocate for their own health, seek timely care, and make informed decisions.

d. Scientific Communication:

- Clear and accessible scientific communication will bridge the gap between researchers, clinicians, and patients.

9. Collaboration and Advocacy

The vision for the future of thymic tumor care relies on collaboration and advocacy:

a. Global Collaboration:

- International collaboration among researchers, clinicians, and patient advocates will drive progress and innovation.

b. Patient Advocacy:

- Patient advocacy organizations will continue to play a pivotal role in raising awareness, supporting patients, and driving research efforts.

c. Policy Advocacy:

- Advocacy for policies that prioritize rare cancer research, access to care, and equitable treatment will shape the future.

d. Research Collaboration:

- Collaborations between academic institutions, pharmaceutical companies, and advocacy groups will fuel breakthroughs in thymic tumor treatment.

10. Conclusion: A Brighter Future for Thymic Tumor Patients

The vision for the future of thymic tumor management is one of hope, progress, and transformation. Through early detection, precision medicine, patient-centered care, global access to care, data-driven decision-making, education, awareness, collaboration, and advocacy, we envision a world where thymic tumors are not only better understood but also more effectively treated. Together, we can work towards a brighter future where thymic tumor patients have improved outcomes, enhanced quality of life, and a renewed sense of hope on their journey towards recovery and survivorship.

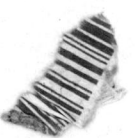

Printed in Great Britain
by Amazon